Q&A Color Review of

Clinical Neurology and Neurosurgery

Guy M. McKhann II MD
Columbia-Presbyterian Medical Center
New York, NY, USA

Neil D. Kitchen MD, FRCS (SN)
The National Hospital for Neurology and Neurosurgery
London, UK

Hadi Manji MD
The National Hospital for Neurology and Neurosurgery
London, UK

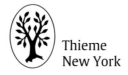

Thieme
New York

First published in the United States of America in 2003 by:
Thieme New York, 333 Seventh Avenue
New York, NY 10001, USA

ISBN 1-58890-154-8

Second impression 2005

Library of Congress Cataloging-in-Publication Data
is available from the publisher

Important note: Medical knowledge is ever-changing. As new research and clinical experience broaden our knowledge, changes in treatment and drug therapy may be required. The authors and editors of the material herein have consulted sources believed to be reliable in their efforts to provide information that is complete and in accord with the standards accepted at the time of publication. However, in view of the possibility of human error by the authors, editors, or publisher of the work herein, or changes in medical knowledge, neither the authors, editors, or publisher, nor any other party who has been involved in the preparation of this work, warrants that the information contained herein is in every respect accurate or complete, and they are not responsible for any errors or omissions or for the results obtained from use of such information. Readers are encouraged to confirm the information contained herein with other sources. For example, readers are advised to check the product information sheet included in the package of each drug they plan to administer to be certain that the information contained in this publication is accurate and that changes have not been made in the recommended dose or in the contraindications for administration. This recommendation is of particular importance in connection with new or infrequently used drugs.

Some of the product names, patents, and registered designs referred to in this book are in fact registered trademarks or proprietary names even though specific reference to this fact is not always made in the text. Therefore, the appearance of a name without designation as proprietary is not to be construed as a representation by the publisher that it is in the public domain.

Copyright © 2003 Manson Publishing Ltd
73 Corringham Road, London NW11 7DL, UK.

Commissioning editor: Jill Northcott
Project manager: Paul Bennett
Printed in Spain

Preface

The clinical neurosciences are an integrated discipline in which physicians (neurologists) and surgeons (neurosurgeons or surgical neurologists) play complementary roles in managing patients. Thus, the questions in this book are spread widely across both specialties, reflecting what the authors feel are common, yet important, clinical problems presenting to the non-specialist.

Neurology is a medical specialty where clinical acumen is still the *sine qua non*. Special investigations then follow and consist primarily of various radiological neuro-imaging studies, EMG and nerve conduction studies, neuropsychology, autonomics, and, increasingly, genetic profiles. Subsequent management includes defining a prognosis and appropriate treatment protocols, some including neurosurgery. In addition, there are primary neurosurgical conditions, such as brain hemorrhage, head injury, and degenerative and traumatic spinal disease. Increasingly, however, the two disciplines work together and patients are managed via a team approach across subspecialty themes – movement disorders, epilepsy, neuro-oncology, brain injury, and peripheral nerve and muscle injury or disease, for example.

Specialists from the United States and the United Kingdom have contributed their experience. Differences in management have more to do with emphasis than resources or fundamental differences in case mix. However, the large number of authors reflects the subspecialization that has occurred in the clinical neurosciences on both sides of the Atlantic. We hope that the reader will find the mix of questions challenging.

Although clinical neuroscience is a fast developing and changing field, we believe that readers will find the contents up-to-date, wide-ranging, informative, and interesting.

Guy M. McKhann II
Neil D. Kitchen
Hadi Manji

3

Contributors

Richard C. Anderson, MD
Columbia University
New York, NY, USA

Anish Bahra, MRCP
The National Hospital for Neurology
and Neurosurgery
London, UK

Alexander Baxter, MD
Beth Israel Medical Center
New York, NY, USA

Kyra Becker, MD
Harborview Medical Center
Seattle, WA, USA

Gary L. Bernardini, MD, PhD
Albany Medical Center
New York, NY, USA

Thomas D. Bird, MD
University of Washington Medical
Center
Seattle, WA, USA

Jeffrey N. Bruce, MD
Columbia University
New York, NY, USA

Jeremy Chataway, MD
The National Hospital for Neurology
and Neurosurgery
London, UK

Katia Cikurel, MD
King's College Hospital
London, UK

Sean Connolly, MD, FRCPI
St Vincent's University Hospital
Dublin, Ireland

E. Sander Connelly Jr, MD
Columbia University
New York, NY, USA

Andrew T. Dailey, MD
University of Utah Medical Center
Salt Lake City, UT, USA

Charles Davie, MD, MRCP
Royal Free Hospital
London, UK

J. Paul Elliott, MD
University of Colorado
Denver, Colo, USA

Neil Feldstein, MD
Columbia University
New York, NY, USA

Magali Fernandez, MD
University of Washington Medical
Center
Seattle, WA, USA

Pamela Freda, MD
Columbia-Presbyterian Medical Center
New York, NY, USA

Neil D. Kitchen, MD, FRCS (SN)
The National Hospital for Neurology
and Neurosurgery
London, UK

Hadi Manji, MA, MD, FRCP
The National Hospital for Neurology
and Neurosurgery
London, UK

John McAuley, MA, MD, MRCP
Royal London Hospital
London, UK

Guy M. McKhann, MD
Columbia-Presbyterian Medical Center
New York, NY, USA

Peter Nestor, MD
Addenbrooke's Hospital
Cambridge, UK

Andrew T. Parsa, MD, PhD
University of California
San Francisco, CA, USA

Mary Reilly, MB, BcH, BAO, MD, MRCPI
The National Hospital for Neurology
and Neurosurgery
London, UK

Jeremy Rees, BSc, MBBS, MRCP, PhD
The National Hospital for Neurology
and Neurosurgery
London, UK

Ali Rezai, MD
Cleveland Clinic Foundation
Cleveland, OH, USA

Paul Riordan-Eva, FRCOphth
Kings College Hospital
London, UK

Peter D. Le Roux, MB, ChB, MD, FACS
The Hospital of the University of
Pennsylvania
Philadelphia, PA, USA

Mathew Walker, MRCP, PhD
The National Hospital for Neurology
and Neurosurgery
London, UK

Thomas T. Warner, MRCP, PhD
Royal Free Hospital
London, UK

Martin Zonenshayn, MD
Weill Medical College of Cornell
University
New York, NY, USA

Abbreviations

ACA anterior cerebral artery
ACAS asymptomatic carotid artery study
ACE acetylcholine esterase
Acom anterior communicating artery
ACTH adrenocorticotrophic hormone
AD Alzheimer's disease
ADCA autosomal dominant cerebellar ataxia
ADEM acute demyelinating encephalomyelitis
ADH antidiuretic hormone
ADM abductor digiti minimi
ADP adenosine diphosphate
AFP alpha fetoprotein
AICA anterior inferior cerebellar artery
AIDS acquired immune deficiency syndrome
AION anterior ischemic optic neuropathy
ALS amyotrophic lateral sclerosis
AP anterior–posterior
APB abductor pollicis brevis
APP amyloid precursor protein
ATLANTIS Alteplase Thrombolysis for Acute Noninterventional Therapy in Ischemic Stroke
ATLS Advanced Trauma Life Support
AVF arteriovenous fistula
AVM arteriovenous malformation

b.i.d. twice daily
BMD Bird muscular dystrophy
BPNH bilateral periventricular nodular heterotopia
BPPV benign paroxymal positional vertigo
BUN blood urea nitrogen

CADASIL cerebral autosomal dominant arteriopathy with subcortical infarcts and leucoencephalopathy
CAPRIE Clopidogrel versus aspirin in patients at risk of ischemic events
CARE cholesterol and recurrent events study
CAST Chinese aspirin study
CBF cerebral blood flow
CEA carotid endarterectomy
Ch choline
CIDP chronic inflammatory demyelinating polyneuropathy
CJD Creutzfeldt–Jakob disease
CMAP compound muscle action potential
$CMRO_2$ cerebral metabolic rate – oxygen
CMT Charcot–Marie–Tooth disease
CMV cytomegalovirus
CNEMG concentric needle electromyography
CNS central nervous system
CPK creatine phosphokinase
CPM central pontine myelinolysis
CPP cerebral perfusion pressure
C-RP C-reactive protein
CRPS complex regional pain syndrome
CSF cerebrospinal fluid
CSR Cheyne-Stokes respiration
CT computerized tomography
CTA computerized tomography angiography
CVP central venous pressure
CXR chest X-ray

DAI diffuse axonal injury
DI diabetes insipidus
DKA diabetes keto acidosis
DMD Duchenne muscular dystrophy
DMES Doppler microembolic signal
DNA deoxyribonucleic acid
DNT dysembryoplastic neuroepithelial tumor

DOPA dihydroxyphenylalanine
DREZ dorsal root entry zone
DRPLA dentatorubral-pallidoluysian atrophy
DWI diffusion weighted imaging

ECA external carotid artery
ECASS European cooperative stroke study
ECG electrocardiography/m
EC–IC external carotid to internal carotid
ECST European carotid surgery trial
EEG electroencephalography
ELITE extreme lateral transcondylar
EMG electromyelography/m
ENT ear nose and throat
EOFAD early-onset familial Alzheimer's disease
ESPS European stroke prevention study
ESR erythrocyte sedimentation rate

FAP familial amyloid polyneuropathy
FBC full blood count
FDG-PET fluoro-deoxy glucose positron emission tomography
FLAIR fluid attenuated inversion recovery
FRDA Friedreich's ataxia
FSHD facioscapulohumeral muscular dystrophy

GCS Glasgow coma scale
GDC Gugliemi detachable coil
GH growth hormone
GM1 anti-ganglioside
GSPN greater superficial petrosal nerve
GSW gunshot wound

HCG human chorionic gonadotropin
HD Huntington's disease
HDL high density lipoprotein
HIV human immunodeficiency virus

HMG-CoA 3-hydroxy-3-methylglutaryl coenzyme A
HMSN hereditary motor and sensory neuropathy

IC internal carotid
ICA internal carotid artery
ICH intracerebral hemorrhage
ICP intracranial pressure
IGF-I insulin-like growth factor I
IgG immunoglobulin G
IIH idiopathic intracranial hypertension
IST International Stroke Trial
i.v. intravenous(ly)

JME juvenile myoclonic epilepsy

LDL low density lipoprotein
LEMS Lambert–Eaton myasthenic syndrome
LIPID long-term intervention with pravastatin in ischemic disease (study)

MAP mean arterial pressure
MCA middle cerebral artery
MI myocardial infarction
MMD myotonic muscular dystrophy
MMNCB multi-focal motor neuropathy with conduction block
MND motor neuron disease
MRA magnetic resonance angiography
MRC Medical Research Council
MRI magnetic resonance imaging
MS multiple sclerosis
MSA multiple system atrophy
MTX methotrexate
MUP motor unit potential

NA N-acetyl aspartate
NASCET North American symptomatic carotid endarterectomy trial
NCEP National cholesterol education program
NCS nerve conduction studies

NCV nerve conduction velocity
NF neurofibromatosis
NIHSS National Institutes of Health stroke scale
NINDS National Institutes of Neurological Disorders and Stroke
NPD Niemann–Pick disease
NPH normal pressure hydrocephalus

OEF oxygen extraction fraction

PAS periodic acid Schiff (stain)
PCA posterior cerebral artery
PCNSL primary CNS lymphoma
Pcom posterior communicating artery
PCR polymerase chain reaction
PCV packed cell volume
PEEP positive end expiratory pressure
PEG percutaneous endoscopic gastrostomy
PET positron emission tomography
PHN post-herpetic neuralgia
PICA posterior inferior cerebellar artery
PLAP placental alkaline phosphatase
PML progressive multifocal leucoencephalopathy
PMP-22 peripheral myelin protein 22
p.o. per os
Po myelin protein zero
PP–MS primary progressive multiple sclerosis

q.d. once daily

RBC red blood cell
rCBF regional cerebral blood flow
RF radiofrequency
RSD reflex sympathetic dystrophy
4S Scandinavian simvastatin survival study
SAH subarachnoid hemorrhage
s.c. subcutaneous
SCA superior cerebellar artery; spinocerebellar ataxia

SCLC small cell lung cancer
SIADH syndrome of inappropriate antidiuretic hormone secretion
SIH spontaneous intracranial hypotension
SNAP sensory nerve action potential
SPECT single positron emission computerized tomography
SSEP somatosensory evoked potential
SSPE subacute sclerosing panencephalitis
SSS superior sagittal sinus

TASS Ticlopidine aspirin stroke study
TB tuberculosis
TCD transcranial Doppler ultrasonography
TENS transcutaneous electrical nerve stimulation
TGN trigeminal neuralgia
TIA transient ischemic attack
TOAST Trial of ORG 10172 in acute stroke treatment
t-PA tissue plasminogen activator
TSC tuberous sclerosis
TTR transthyretin-related

UO urine output

VA vertebral artery
VER visual evoked responses
VGCC voltage gated calcium channels

WASIDS Warfarin-aspirin symptomatic intracranial disease study
WBC white blood cell

ZN Ziehl–Neelsen (stain)

Classification of cases

Cerebral blood flow 20, 71, 107, 111, 141

Cerebrovascular disease, malformations and aneurysms 12, 17, 29, 36, 39, 52, 54, 58, 59, 74, 77, 93, 110, 119, 157, 172, 180

Coma/unconsciousness 2, 5, 94, 107, 141, 155

Congenital and inherited disorders 12, 22, 26, 44, 50, 60, 64, 65, 66, 82, 87, 98, 103, 119, 124

Degenerative disorders 13, 24, 25, 38, 42, 78, 99, 104, 121, 143, 162

Epilepsy 45, 50, 53, 64, 118, 152, 160, 171

Facial pain and pain syndromes 10, 18, 32, 49, 57, 73, 135, 178, 108

Head/brain injury 144, 5, 41, 81, 141, 170

Headache and migraine 119, 1, 23, 46, 68, 100, 165

Hydrocephalus 6, 7, 40, 67, 101, 128, 169

Infective and inflammatory disorders 9, 19, 33, 70, 76, 85, 86, 88, 102, 112, 114, 140, 146, 148, 156, 159, 164

Intracranial hemorrhage 3, 6, 7, 17, 29, 40, 46, 74, 80, 93, 110, 123, 163

Intracranial pressure 68, 92, 123, 137, 173

Intracranial tumors 43, 50, 53, 56, 66, 97, 99, 113, 118, 125, 131, 158, 169, 179

Malignancy, manifestations of 14, 105, 129, 144, 158

Movement disorders 13, 16, 26, 28, 37, 44, 55, 83, 84, 115, 116, 132, 133

Neuroectodermal syndromes 22, 34, 66, 87, 177

Operative/anesthetic complications 30, 69, 71, 79, 111

Ophthalmic/visual symptoms 15, 22, 54, 75, 87, 91, 113, 117, 137, 144

Peripheral nerve disorders 8, 11, 21, 31, 47, 60, 65, 72, 98, 136, 138, 167, 168, 175, 176

Pituitary and hypothalamic lesions 35, 61, 95, 96, 109, 122, 126, 127

Skull lesion 4

Spinal injury and disease 8, 11, 63, 72, 85, 86, 89, 90, 134, 142, 124, 139, 159, 175, 176

Voluntary muscle disorders 27, 48, 62, 82, 91, 103, 130, 161

Picture acknowledgements

58, 59, 193a–d Courtesy of Dr A. Baxter
82, 103 Copyright © 1971 Medcom, Inc, New York, USA
165 Courtesy of Dr N. Silver
166 Courtesy of Dr N. Murray
174b Courtesty of Dr T. Revesz
177c Copyright © 1998 Current Medicine, Inc, Philadelphia, USA

1 This 67-year-old male presents with a 5-week history of severe left-sided retro-orbital pain which radiates to the upper teeth, jaw and cheek (1). He complains of a dull background pain at all times with excruciating exacerbations lasting between 1–2 hours up to three times a day. He describes the same symptoms occurred for several weeks 1 and 3 years previously.

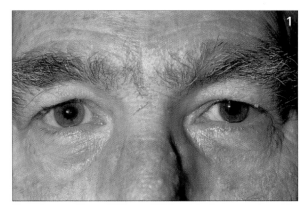

i. What is the diagnosis?
ii. What other clinical features in the history would support the diagnosis?
iii. What treatment would you offer the patient?

2 A 35-year-old chronic alcoholic was admitted to hospital comatose. Investigations revealed a serum sodium of 100 mmol/L (100 mEq/L). The patient's neurologic condition improved with correction of her sodium level. However, 1 week later her neurologic condition deteriorated again. On examination she was alert and oriented. She required ventilatory support. Eye movements revealed a horizontal gaze palsy bilaterally with normal vertical eye movements. There was evidence of lower motor neuron bilateral facial weakness. There was grade 2 power in the limbs with a pyramidal distribution of weakness. Reflexes were all pathologically brisk with bilateral extensor plantars. The MRI is an axial proton density weighted scan without contrast through the level of the pons (2).

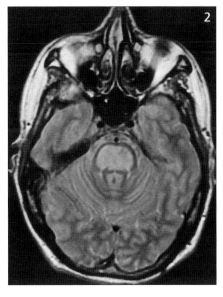

i. What is the most likely explanation for her comatose state on admission?
ii. What abnormality is shown in the MRI scan?
iii. What neurologic complication did she develop?
iv. Why may this have occurred?

1 i. This man has a left-sided partial Horner's syndrome. The diagnosis is cluster headache.

ii. Although the pain experienced is predominantly retro-orbital and temporal, almost half of patients experience pain radiating down to the cheek, jaw and teeth. Unlike migraine, patients are restless during the attacks and movement does not exacerbate the pain. The pain is accompanied with ipsilateral autonomic features. Most commonly these include lacrimation, conjunctival injection, nasal congestion and rhinorrhea, and less commonly a partial Horner's syndrome which can persist between headaches. The attacks tend to last 15–180 minutes and can occur up to eight times a day, characteristically awaking the patient during the night about 1.5–2 hours after falling asleep. The attacks can occur daily in bouts which usually last 1–3 months. Patients tend to experience a bout every 1–2 years; however, the longest reported remission period has been 30 years. Ten to 20% have chronic symptoms with attacks occurring for >1 year without significant remission periods (currently defined as a 2–week period). Characteristically, during a bout attacks can be triggered by alcohol. The peak age of onset is between the 3rd and 4th decade. Symptomatic cluster headache has been reported in patients with pituitary tumors, anterior circulation aneurysms, meningioma of the high cervical canal and vertebral artery dissection. Patients presenting with their first episode should be investigated.

iii. The most effective abortive treatments for cluster headache are subcutaneous sumatriptan and 100% oxygen at a flow rate of at least 7 L/min. The most effective prophylactic agents include verapamil, methysergide, lithium, and corticosteroids as a short-term adjunctive measure.

2 i. It is likely that this patient had developed an inappropriate secretion of ADH (SIADH) resulting in coma. Rapid correction of hyponatremia is a well recognized precipitant of central pontine myelinosis (CPM).

ii. The MRI scan shows a diffuse increase of signal within the pons consistent with diagnosis.

iii. CPM is an acute demyelinating pathology most frequently seen with rapid alteration of sodium levels in the context of alcoholism or malnutrition. The demyelinating lesion in CPM as the name implies is normally confined to the pons, with a rim of intact myelin between the lesion and the surface of the thalamus, striatum and lateral geniculate bodies. The disorder has also been reported in association with Wernicke's disease, carcinoma and severe burns, the latter particularly observed in children. CPM can present as a 'locked-in syndrome'. Treatment is supportive. Unfortunately, in those patients developing severe neurologic deficit the incidence of mortality is ~90%.

iv. CPM secondary to rapid correction of hyponatremia in a patient with SIADH.

3 An elderly right-handed male was noted by his wife to develop progressive confusion over a week. He started having word finding difficulties and demonstrated deterioration in his handwriting and subsequent right-sided weakness. He was subsequently admitted to hospital.

i. What are the possible etiologies for his symptoms?

ii. Describe the findings on his head CT (3).

iii. What are the important aspects of his history?

iv. What is the proper treatment and what is his prognosis?

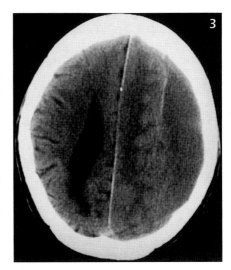

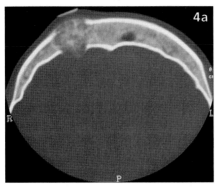

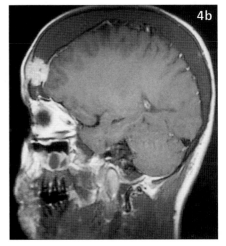

4 These scans (4a, b) show a rapidly enlarging mass on the forehead of a 24-year-old male.

i. What are the investigations and what do they show?

ii. What is the underlying condition?

iii. What is the differential diagnosis of the skull lesion?

3 i. The patient's neurologic symptoms and signs indicate a left-sided brain lesion involving speech and motor areas. This may result from stroke, a tumor with surrounding edema, or other space occupying region such as hemorrhage.

ii. The head CT show an extra-axial lesion isodense with brain with mass effect. There is minimal acute blood layered inferiorly. This is consistent with a chronic subdural hematoma.

iii. Many elderly patients develop chronic subdural hematomas after a previous fall which they considered insignificant and from which they were initially asymptomatic.

iv. If the mass effect is minimal, some chronic subdural hematomas may be treated conservatively. In symptomatic patients or those with significant mass effect, the initial treatment is burr hole drainage. The typical appearance of chronic subdural blood is described as 'crank-case oil'. Sometimes repeat drainage procedures are required due to rebleeding of vascularized membranes that may form within hematomas that bleed multiple times. The prognosis is usually good.

4 i. Scan **4a** is a CT brain scan – bony windows. A medullary mass is shown which expands and erodes both cortices. Scan **4b** is a sagittal T1 MRI with gadolinium. The mass enhances. The grossly abnormal skull is also shown, indicating thickened, active marrow.

ii. Thalassemia major.

iii. The skull lesion was biopsied. Pathology indicated focal medullary extrapoiesis. No specific other treatment was recommended apart from curettage. Recurrent enlargement may respond to focal radiotherapy. This is an unusual site for focal extrapoiesis which classically occurs in the ribs. Other pre-operative possibilities included lymphoma, leukemia and hemangioma.

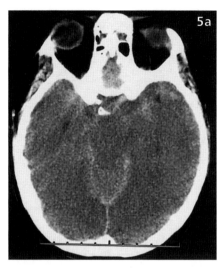
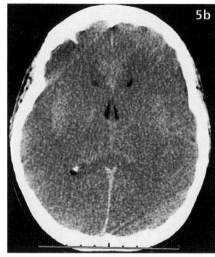

5 A 36-year-old female suffered a cardiorespiratory arrest after sedation for a minor procedure. She was successfully resuscitated but remained comatose for several days. The CT scans (5a, b) were obtained 3 days after her respiratory arrest.
i. What are the findings?
ii. What is the patient's prognosis for neurologic recovery?

6 A 52-year-old male presented to the emergency department complaining of new-onset headache beginning yesterday. Although he suffers from chronic headaches this one came on suddenly and is described as the worst headache of his life. The usual pain killers are not working. On examination, he is alert, complaining of severe headache. A non-contrast CT scan was obtained (6).

What is the diagnosis and what are the possible causes?

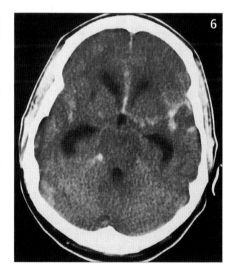

5 i. The CT images (5a, b) show loss of the normal difference in CT attenuation between gray and white matter. The basal ganglia and cerebral cortex, which are normally sharply defined, are indistinguishable from the adjacent white matter. The sylvian fissures, cortical sulci, and perimesencephalic cisterns are compressed, reflecting diffuse cerebral swelling. A CT scan obtained at the time of cardiorespiratory arrest (5c), is normal.

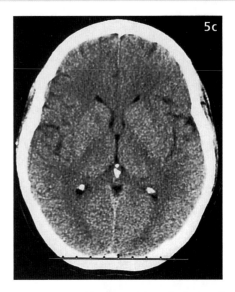

Hypoxic/ischemic injury to the brain can result from inadequate blood oxygenation (carbon monoxide poisoning, near drowning, and respiratory arrest), systemic hypoperfusion (cardiac arrest, cardiac tamponade, and anaphylaxis), increased ICP (head trauma, cerebral infarct with edema), or histiotoxic insults (hypoglycemia and cyanide). CT findings are often initially normal but findings of cerebral edema and loss of gray–white definition may develop within hours. In less severe cases, decreased CT attenuation may be seen in the globi pallidi, putamina, medial temporal lobes, and border zones between cerebral arterial territories.

ii. The prognosis for patients with complete loss of cerebral anatomic definition and sulcal effacement 3 days following hypoxic ischemic injury is dismal, with most survivors remaining in a persistent vegetative state.

6 He has suffered a SAH and has evidence of hydrocephalus. There is a predominance of blood in the left sylvian fissure suggesting that the source may be in that region. The most common causes of SAH are: (1) trauma (this patient has no such history); (2) a ruptured intracerebral aneurysm; (3) a ruptured AVM (with which there is usually evidence of an intracerebral parenchymal hemorrhage as well or flow voids on the CT scan). Other less likely causes include: vasculitides, tumor, arterial dissection, disorders of coagulation, dural sinus thrombosis, dural AVF, spinal AVM and pituitary apoplexy.

The hydrocephalus is undoubtedly secondary to the SAH and is the result of blood interfering with CSF reabsorption either by blocking the ventricular outlet system or drainage through the arachnoid granulations. Hydrocephalus is seen on 15% of admission CT scans for SAH with nearly half of these patients experiencing additional symptoms from the hydrocephalus.

7 With regard to the patient in 6:
i. If the CT scan had been negative, what would have been the next diagnostic maneuver?
ii. Given that the CT scan is positive what is the next test you should order, and should some other intervention be employed prior to that test being performed?

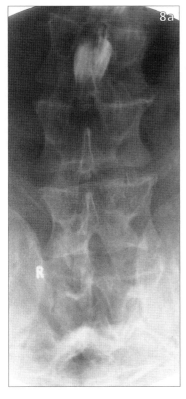

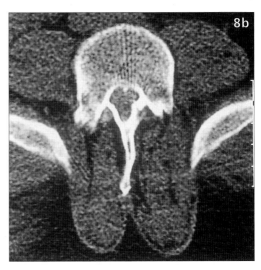

8 This short statured individual suffers severe bilateral leg pains on minimal walking.
i. What do these investigations show (8a, b)?
ii. What is the underlying condition?
iii. What treatment was performed?

7, 8: Answers

7 i. If the CT scan had been negative, a lumbar puncture should be performed. Failure to do so may result in missing a SAH. Retrospective studies show that missing the diagnosis at this juncture is responsible for the greatest amount of preventable morbidity associated with this disease. This patient is currently in grade II condition, severe headache only, and is likely to have a good outcome (90% chance). If he is sent home and re-presents in worse condition from a rebleed (grade III [mild focal deficit or confusion], grade IV [stupor, moderate hemiparesis or early posturing], or grade V [deep coma with advanced posturing]) it is much less likely that his outcome will be good (70% grade III, 40% grade IV, 5% grade V). The lumbar puncture most likely will demonstrate an opening elevated pressure, and non-clotting bloody fluid that does not clear with sequential tubes. Xanthochromia which results from delayed breakdown of blood products may take 24–48 hours to develop, but can be seen as early as 6 hours in 70% of patients. This finding is helpful in differentiating a SAH from a traumatic tap and can be easily performed at the bedside by placing one tube upright for 10–15 minutes and examining the supernate. In true cases of SAH the cell count should usually exceed 100 000 RBC/mm^3 and there should be >2 WBC for each RBC (i.e. usually >200 WBC/mm^3 in SAH). The protein is also usually elevated.

ii. Given the CT scan shown, there is no need to perform a lumbar puncture for confirmation. In fact, such a procedure risks increasing the transmural pressure across an aneurysm (which is the most likely cause) and has been linked to an increased incidence of early rebleeding. Similarly, although the patient has marked hydrocephalus, placing an externalized ventricular drain is only indicated in those patients with evidence of stupor on examination as this maneuver may precipitate rebleeding. The next test to order after sending routine blood work (including coagulation parameters) is a four-vessel cerebral angiogram. This is the gold standard for diagnosing a cerebral aneurysm which is the most dangerous cause of SAH, requiring immediate attention. As 30% of patients with aneurysmal SAH will harbor greater than one aneurysm all four vessels must be visualized. The only reason to forego an angiogram is in a patient presenting with signs of acute herniation from an associated intracerebral hematoma which requires emergent evacuation. In such cases an infusion CT scan or CTA can often demonstrate the aneurysm responsible. (See also 17.)

8 i. Myelography and CT scanning show two features: lumbar canal stenosis with blockage of contrast flow. Extreme muscle hypertrophy is also seen.
ii. Achondroplasic dwarfism causing lumbar canal stenosis. Such individuals can suffer whole spine stenosis.
iii. Decompressive lumbar laminectomy was performed. Surgery is complicated by the excessive muscle bulk and the exaggerated lumbar lordosis.

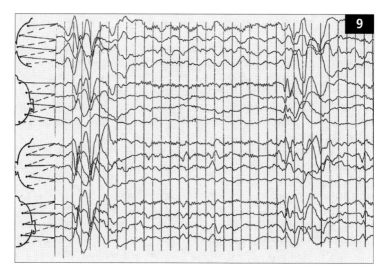

9 This EEG was recorded from a 13-year-old female with a 4-week history of abrupt jerks in all limbs, followed by slow return to resting position (9). Over the previous 3 months, school performance had deteriorated. The EEG pattern persisted throughout waking and sleeping states.
i. What abnormality is shown?
ii. What is the likely diagnosis?
iii. What other investigations would help to confirm the diagnosis?

10 A 28-year-old female complains of a 2-week history of a heavy feeling in the left side of her face, accompanied by constant throbbing and aching pain. It is more severe in the mornings and evenings, and is significantly exacerbated by lowering the head while bending down. Carbamazepine is prescribed but the patient calls back several days later stating that now, in addition to the pain, she has foul-smelling nasal discharge.
i. What is the cause of this patient's facial pain?
ii. What is the differential diagnosis of facial pain?

9 i. There are bilateral polyphasic sharp- and slow-wave complexes of high amplitude, occurring at intervals of approximately 4 seconds. These discharges last up to 2 seconds. The background EEG between discharges is grossly abnormal, particularly on the left side where irregular theta and delta slowing is evident.
ii. This pattern of abnormality persisted in a periodic pattern, including during sleep, and the complexes remained remarkably stereotyped. They could be evoked by tactile stimuli, and were usually accompanied by a visible jerk of all limbs. The typical EEG changes of sleep were not present. These EEG features are virtually diagnostic of the intermediate stage of SSPE.
iii. CSF analysis. The CSF contained antibody to measles virus in high concentration. CSF gammaglobulin may also be raised.

10 i. The patient described has the hallmark symptoms of acute maxillary sinusitis. The pain is generally depicted as throbbing, present over one or more sinuses, continuous rather than paroxysmal, and is worsened by downward positioning of the head. There is often an accompanying foul-smelling nasal discharge as a result of the infection. Tenderness and/or erythema of the cheek aids in the diagnosis. Treatment consists of antibiotics and decongestants, or in cases where a fistula is present, surgical enlargement of the fistula to allow drainage of infected contents. Of note, other facial sinuses, such as the frontal, ethmoid, and sphenoid sinuses, may be involved as well.
ii. The differential diagnosis of facial pain is rather extensive. It includes vascular conditions (migraine, temporal arteritis), malignancies affecting the sinuses or the trigeminal ganglion, ophthalmic conditions (glaucoma, optic neuritis), and dental conditions. In a study of 1,100 patients with TGN, one-third had unnecessary tooth extractions prior to being diagnosed correctly.

The remainder of the differential diagnosis consists of other types of neuralgia, such as glossopharyngeal neuralgia, PHN, and cluster headaches. Glossopharyngeal neuralgia is very rare (incidence of 5 per million) and is characterized by repeated bouts of severe sharp/shooting pain in the distribution of the ninth cranial nerve (tonsillar area and throat radiating to eye, ear, nose, and shoulder). PHN is described as severe constant burning pain with sharp exacerbations, often accompanied by allodynia (sensation of pain resulting from a normally painless sensory stimulus). The pain occurs after a bout of acute facial herpes zoster and is commonly unilateral in the V1 distribution. V1 distribution pain in TGN, on the other hand, occurs in only 2% of affected patients. Cluster headaches typically affect young men who tend to be anxious, and possess a more aggressive personality. The bouts of headaches, typically lasting 30 minutes to 2 hours, are cyclic and the timing of the next attack can often be predicted by the patient. Typically, the attacks occur daily for 1–2 months, with periods of remission for 6–18 months. Ingestion of alcohol may precipitate an attack.

11 A far lateral disc herniation at the L4–5 level could cause the following except:
(a) Loss of patellar reflex.
(b) Weakness of foot dorsiflexion.
(c) Weakness of knee extension.
(d) Weakness of extension of the first toe.
(e) Sensory loss in the calf.

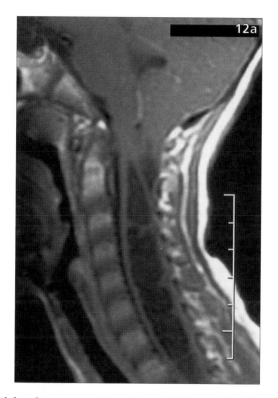

12 A 14-year-old female presents with a 6-month history of neck pain and intermittent numbness and tingling in her fingers. Recently, she noticed some difficulty with swallowing. Her MRI is shown (**12a**).
i. What is the diagnosis?
ii. What are the treatment options?
iii. Discuss the pathophysiology of this condition.

11 (d). The nerve root affected by a far lateral disc herniation is that which has already exited the neural foramen at that level. In this case the affected root is the L4 root. The only muscle group listed that does not have a component of L4 innervation is the extensor hallicus longus (L5–S1).

12 i. This patient has a Chiari I malformation with associated hydrosyringomyelia. Chiari I is characterized by caudal displacement of the cerebellar tonsils at least 3–5 mm (0.1–0.2 in) below the foramen magnum. Hydrosyringomyelia occurs in 20–30% of cases. Patients with Chiari I malformations present clinically with symptoms and signs of: (1) brainstem compression at the foramen magnum; (2) hydrocephalus; or (3) syringomyelia. Chiari II malformation, on the other hand, is characterized by a caudally dislocated cervicomedullary junction, pons, fourth ventricle, and medulla. They are often associated with myelomeningocele, hydrocephalus, beaking of the tectum, absence of septum pellucidum, and medullary kinking.

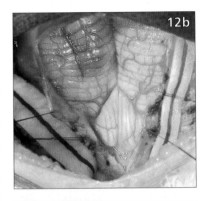

ii. Patients respond best when operated on within 2 years of the onset of symptoms, so early surgery is recommended for symptomatic patients. Although in the past the syrinx was often treated directly with fenestration or shunting, the most frequently performed operation now is a suboccipital decompression (**12b**) with cervical laminectomy of C1 through C2 or C3. Many neurosurgeons include dural patch grafting (**12c**), and some advocate arachnoid dissection with separation of the cerebellar tonsils.

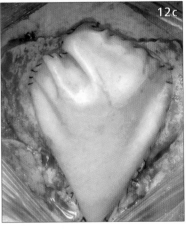

iii. Chiari I malformations are associated with communicating syringomyelia, or a primary dilatation of the central canal. There are three prevailing theories of syrinx formation: (1) the hydrodynamic (water-hammer) theory of Gardner claims that systolic pulsations are transmitted with each heartbeat from the intracranial cavity to the central canal; (2) Williams' theory suggests that maneuvers raising CSF pressure (coughing, valsalva and so on) cause hydrodissection through the spinal cord tissue; and (3) the Oldfield theory claims that the syrinx is created by transmission of increased venous pressure.

13 A 45-year-old male with chorea and cognitive difficulties has the head CT scan shown here (13). His mother died at a nursing home, from a progressive neurologic disease. His uncle is in a mental institution.
i. What does the CT scan show?
ii. What is the most likely diagnosis?
iii. What is the most useful test to confirm the clinical diagnosis?

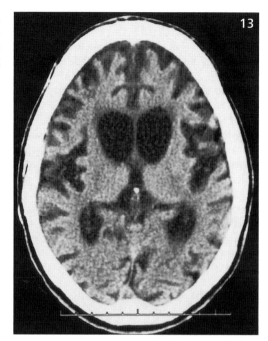

14 A 74-year-old female presented with a rapid decline of memory over a 2-month period. Bedside cognitive testing revealed preserved attention and concentration. There was no language disturbance, short term memory was severely impaired. General examination was normal. Neurologic examination only revealed stimulus sensitive myoclonus.
i. Where is the abnormality on the MRI scan (14)?
ii. What is the differential diagnosis?
iii. What antibody tests are indicated?
iv. What other investigations should be performed?

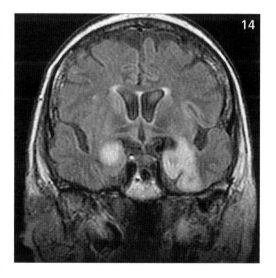

13 i. The CT shows marked bilateral caudate atrophy and diffuse cortical atrophy.

ii. This patient has HD. HD is a neurodegenerative disorder characterized by involuntary movements, cognitive, and behavioral disturbances. There are adventitious movements and difficulties with the motor control of voluntary movements. The behavioral dysfunction presents with problems in planning, initiating, and completing tasks. Psychiatric disturbances can be the presenting symptoms. The average age at onset is 35–45 years, but onset can vary from childhood to old age. It is an autosomal dominant genetic disease. In this patient, the history of chorea, cognitive difficulties, and a family history of neurologic problems is very suggestive of HD.

iii. There is a commercially available and highly specific DNA test. The gene for HD is on chromosome 4p16. The disorder is caused by an expansion of a CAG trinucleotide repeat in the HD gene. The normal repeat range is 6–27. Greater than 38 repeats is abnormal and will lead to symptoms of HD during a normal life span. The 36–38 repeat range is an intermediate one in which patients may or may not develop symptoms but their children are at risk for the disease. In the 28–35 repeat range patients will not develop symptoms, but their children are at risk for inheriting a larger expansion. The test detects the number of repeats in the HD gene. A positive test together with the clinical picture and the family history confirms the diagnosis.

14 i. The MRI scan shows high T2 signal in the mesial temporal lobe bilaterally, more on the left than right. This involves the uncus, amygdala and also the hippocampus.

ii. The radiological differential diagnosis is either herpes simplex encephalitis or a paraneoplastic limbic encephalitis. The time course favors the latter diagnosis.

iii. Paraneoplastic limbic encephalitis may be associated with anti-Hu (SCLC) and anti-Ma2 (testis) antibodies.

iv. Apart from a thorough physical examination it would be appropriate to do the following: chest X-ray; mammogram; abdominal ultrasound. FDG-PET scanning may also be helpful in the detection of occult neoplasms where the screening tests are negative.

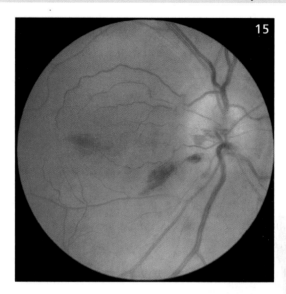

15 A 70-year-old female presented with unilateral acute visual loss, associated with an inferior altitudinal field defect and a swollen optic disc (15).
i. What is the diagnosis?
ii. How should the patient be managed?

16 A 40-year-old right-handed male presents with 10 years of intermittent tremor of the hands, most notably occurring when he pours out drinks on special occasions. The tremor settles after a few drinks. He is asthmatic and he feels his inhaler may also precipitate the tremor. There is no family history of tremor or other neurologic disease. On examination, he has a fine rapid tremor when holding his arms outstretched and a slight 'yes–yes' direction titubation (head tremor). There are no other abnormal findings.
i. What is the likely diagnosis?
ii. Give an important differential diagnosis.
iii. What are the management options?

15 i. The diagnosis is AION. The optic disc is not only swollen but also has a number of superficial hemorrhages.

ii. It is essential that giant cell arteritis is excluded. The patient should be specifically questioned about symptoms of temporal arteritis (e.g. headache, scalp tenderness, and jaw claudication) and polymyalgia rheumatica. The superficial temporal arteries should be palpated for tenderness and the presence of a normal pulse. An urgent ESR and/or C-RP should be performed (jaw claudication, ESR >45 mm/hour, and C-RP >25 g/L are particularly strong indicators of giant cell arteritis). If there is suspicion of giant cell arteritis, high dose systemic steroids (oral prednisolone 1–1.5 mg/kg/day, preceded by i.v. methylprednisolone 1 g/day for 3 days if there is bilateral visual loss) should be started immediately and a temporal artery biopsy arranged to confirm the diagnosis. In cases of non-arteritic AION, the major predisposing factor is congenitally small optic discs, but risk factors for arteriosclerosis such as systemic hypertension, diabetes mellitus, and hyperlipidemia need to be identified. There is a risk of fellow eye involvement in non-arteritic AION, which may be reduced by low dose aspirin therapy.

16 i. Essential tremor. This commonly-occurring tremor characteristically occurs bilaterally during postural tasks. There may be a family history of similar tremor. The tremor is generally relieved by relatively modest quantities of alcohol. Progression may occur over many years from young adulthood onward and it may take some time for essential tremor to become a sufficient nuisance for patients to seek medical attention. However, more severely affected individuals may become disabled by a coarse slower tremor that also appears at rest and is superimposed upon movement. The pathophysiology of essential tremor remains unclear but may relate to abnormal neuronal oscillatory activity in cerebello-thalamic pathways.

ii. Enhanced physiologic tremor of hyperthyroidism. Enhanced physiologic tremor simply describes the situation where the normal tremor manifest in all individuals becomes of large enough amplitude to become a nuisance. Typical factors that augment physiologic tremor include advancing age, fatigue and adrenergic stimulation, although it must be noted that such factors also exacerbate primarily pathogenic tremors such as essential tremor. Adrenergic stimulation accounts for the tremor experienced during anxiety and in hyperthyroidism or on taking beta-agonists for asthma. It is thus important to search for associated features of hyperthyroidism and to test thyroid function in any patient with a fine bilateral postural tremor.

iii. A mild essential tremor may be best dealt with by simply explaining the nature of the condition to the patient. Given its slowly progressive nature, a young individual with essential tremor may be advised to avoid careers in professions requiring fine hand control. As a result of its efficacy in relieving tremor, alcoholism may also become a problem. Medication includes the barbiturate primidone, best given in syrup form which allows introduction of very small doses (c. 25 mg) to avoid somnolent side effects, and beta-blockers such as slow release propranolol. A recently established treatment for severe disabling cases is deep brain lesioning or stimulation, generally in the ventro-intermediate nucleus of the thalamus.

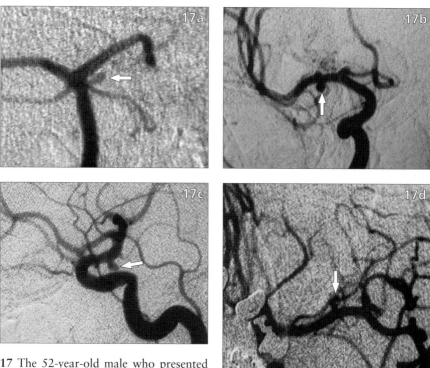

17 The 52-year-old male who presented in 6, 7 underwent four vessel cerebral angiography. Shown are: the right vertebral AP injection (17a), the right ICA AP injection (17b), the left ICA lateral injection (17c), and the left ICA base view injection (17d).

i. Identify the lesions on each injection (arrows).

ii. Which lesion most likely bled and what criteria are used to reach this decision?

iii. What procedure would you recommend and why?

iv. What would you recommend be done for the remaining lesions given the fact that he makes a full recovery from this episode of bleeding, and why?

17 i. The vertebral injection shows neither PICA origin or the vertebrobasilar junction to satisfaction, but there is a left SCA aneurysm. The right ICA injection shows an M1 segment aneurysm with a branch coming out of its base; additional view would be necessary to rule out other lesions, but when they were done no other lesions were identified and the fullness at the A1 takeoff was shown to be a loop. The left lateral injection shows a Pcom aneurysm and the left ICA base view demonstrates what appears to be a MCA bifurcation aneurysm.

ii. The lesion which was most likely to have bled in order is: (1) left MCA; (2) left Pcom; (3) left SCA; (4) right MCA. The best predictor is the location of the bleed which in this case favors a left-sided lesion, particularly one in the sylvian fissure. However, many midline lesions will show laterally placed subarachnoid blood probably because the patient fell to that side during the ictus. Perhaps the most significant localizing patterns are when there is significant interhemispheric blood. This predicts an Acom aneurysm if present. The other pattern is one in which the blood is isolated to the posterior fossa. This may occur with Pcom aneurysms but rarely with any other anterior circulation lesion. Other predictors in order of importance are: (1) aneurysm size; (2) presence of dome irregularity; (3) evidence of local spasm. Midline lesions and posterior fossa lesions bleed more commonly than lateralized or anterior circulation lesions.

iii. Given the likelihood that the left MCA or Pcom aneurysm bled, the most reasonable course of action would be to perform a left pterional craniotomy and clip each of the left-sided lesions starting with the MCA and proceeding to the Pcom and SCA afterwards. Some surgeons might prefer to leave the SCA aneurysm untreated, given the degree of retraction necessary on the dominant temporal lobe in the acute setting. If a left-sided exploration were negative a contralateral craniotomy could be performed at the same sitting to address the contralateral lesion. The decision for direct clipping rather than GDC embolization for this patient is based on the fact that each of these aneurysms is small and favorably situated. The patient is young and in good condition and is likely to have a good outcome with lasting cure from direct surgical management. GDC would be more appropriate for an elderly patient in poor medical condition with an unfavorably situated lesion. As GDC treatment cannot assess which aneurysm actually bled it would require all left-sided aneurysms to be treated, and thus would offer less in the way of procedural risk reduction.

iv. In fact, the left MCA aneurysm had bled and the left Pcom was clipped in the acute period as it was easily accessible. The residual risk posed by the <1 cm (<0.4 in) left SCA and right M1 aneurysms would have to be considered to each be in the order of about 1% per year. Given that 75% of patients suffering SAH suffer permanent morbidity or mortality, the lifetime risk would be:

$$1 - (\text{percent without an event})^{\text{years of life left}} = 1 - 0.98^{25} = 43\%.$$

Thus, treatment of the unruptured lesions makes sense if it can be accomplished with a combined morbidity of <10%. This of course assumes complete protection afforded by the treatment. As there is little evidence at present that GDC actually results in long-term cure of most aneurysms, either observation or surgery makes the most sense. If surgery on the SCA is to be considered it should be performed about 1 month after the bleed to ensure that spasm and swelling have resolved but to minimize the scar tissue formation.

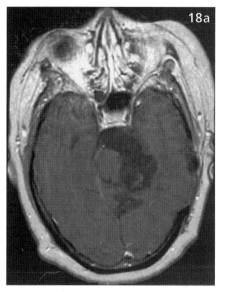
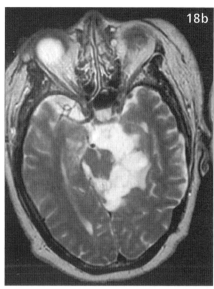

18 A 45-year-old female developed left-sided lower facial pain. **18a, b** were obtained as part of an MRI examination.
i. Which MRI sequences are shown?
ii. Where is the lesion located and what are its signal characteristics?
iii. What is the likely diagnosis?

19 At the age of 30 years, this male developed weight loss and diarrhea. Two years later he presented with memory problems, hypersomnolescence, ataxia and slurred speech. Examination showed impairment of short term memory, slow horizontal and vertical saccades, a supranuclear gaze palsy and palatal myoclonus. A CSF examination revealed: 24 mm^3 lymphocytes; protein 1.79 g/L (0.18 g/dl); and sugar 3.2 mmol/L (57.7 mg/dl). Blood sugar 4.8 mmol/L (86.5 mg/dl).
i. What abnormality is shown on the MRI scan (**19**)?
ii. What other non-neurologic investigation may be necessary?
iii. Are there any other tests that can be performed on the CSF?
iv. What is the treatment?

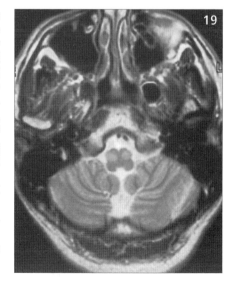

18 i. The images are T1-weighted (**18a**) and T2-weighted (**18b**) sequences using the spin-echo technique. On a T1-weighted image, gray matter is lower in signal intensity than white matter, fat is bright, and CSF is dark. On a true T2-weighted image, gray matter is higher in signal intensity than white matter, CSF is bright and fat is dark. On newer, fast spin-echo T2 sequences, fat and CSF are both bright. T1 sequences demonstrate anatomy well and serve as background when MRI contrast agents are used. T2 sequences show many focal pathologic lesions as areas of high signal, including primary and metastatic tumors, infarcts, demyelination, cerebritis, and abscesses.
ii. This lesion involves the left suprasellar, crural, ambient, and quadrigeminal plate cisterns. It is definitely extra-axial (outside the brain parenchyma), and displaces the midbrain to the right. The patient's symptoms are due to compression of the second and third divisions of the trigeminal nerve, which is surrounded by this lesion. Its signal characteristics are similar, but not identical to CSF: dark on T1- and T2-weighted Images.
iii. The likely diagnosis is epidermoid. These are benign, slowly growing masses that arise from epithelial elements that remain within the cranium after neural tube closure. Epidermoids can occur in the cerebellopontine angle, sella and parasellar regions, perimesencephalic cisterns and fourth ventricle. Occasionally they are seen in the diploic space of the skull or the middle ear as erosive bony lesions. Differential diagnostic considerations include: arachnoid cyst, racemose cysticercosis, craniopharyngioma, and dermoid.

19 i. The MRI scan shows high signal in the mid brain area – Mollarett's triangle – which is the site of lesion to account for palatal myoclonus.
ii. The history of gastrointestinal symptoms suggest that a duodenal biopsy should be performed. In particular, two conditions that may be related to the neurologic illness are celiac disease and Whipple's disease. For the latter, macrophages containing PAS positive rod shaped organisms may be found in biopsy material. PCR can be used to isolate the organism *Tropheryma whippelii*. Villous atrophy helps to make a diagnosis of celiac disease. Anti-gliaden antibodies may be present in the sera of patients with celiac disease.
iii. The same PCR technique can be used to identify *T. whippelii* in the CSF.
iv. The antibiotic regimen suggested includes at least 2 weeks of i.v. treatment with penicillin and streptomycin followed by long term cotrimoxazole for 1–2 years. The alternative is to use of the third generation cephalosporins such as ceftriaxone i.v. for 1 month followed by 2 years of oral cefixime.

20 The diagram illustrates the mechanism of cerebral auto-regulation, which controls CBF in the face of changing blood pressure (**20**).

Is the shift in the curve to the right (solid arrow) caused by:
(a) hyperthyroidism
(b) hypocalcemia
(c) hypertension
(d) hypotension?

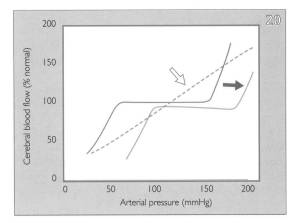

21 A 43-year-old male gave a 2-year history of feeling dizzy in bed. This occurred when he lay back in bed but also when he rolled to the right but not to the left. There were no symptoms of tinnitus or hearing loss. Five years previously he had been involved in a road traffic accident, and had suffered a mild head injury. Neurologic examination was normal.
i. What is the most likely diagnosis based on the history?
ii. What specific neuro-otological test should be carried out?
iii. What are the diagnostic features of this test in the condition this patient suffers from?
iv. What are the treatments available for this condition?

22 A 29-year-old female presented to an ophthalmologist with bilateral painless visual loss, worse in the right eye (down to counting fingers). She had also noticed increasing deafness in the right ear and unsteadiness of gait. On examination she had bilateral optic atrophy, a left partial third and fourth nerve palsy and bilateral sensorineural deafness, worse on the right than the left.
i. What does the CT scan (**22**) show?
ii. How can the other neurologic problems be accounted for?
iii. What is the most likely underlying condition?

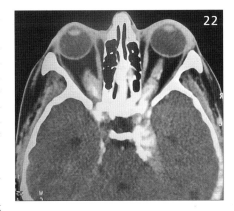

20 (c). Cerebral autoregulation represents a mechanism by which the brain maintains CBF over a wide range of blood pressure. A rightward shift in the curve (solid arrow) occurs in patients with long-standing hypertension. Thus, overexuberant lowering of blood pressure with anti-hypertensives beyond the lower limit of the shifted auto-regulation curve may result in cerebral hypoperfusion not seen in normotensives at the same level of blood pressure. With failed autoregulation, cerebral perfusion becomes linear and directly related to increases in blood pressure (open arrow and dotted line).

21 i. The diagnosis is BPPV. This is due to the presence of debris, most commonly in the posterior semicircular canal (canalolithiasis). Predisposing factors include previous head injury, previous episodes of labyrinthitis presumed viral, prolonged bed rest for any reason, vertobasilar ischemia, and increasing age.
ii. The Hallpike test.
iii. In BPPV, the features of a positive Hallpike test include the following. (1) Latency: vertigo and nystagmus begin 1 or more seconds after the head is tilted toward the affected ear. (2) Duration: less than 1 minute and gradually reduces after 10–40 seconds. (3) Nystagmus: this is linear rotatory with the fast phase beating towards the undermost ear (geotrophic). When the patient returns to a seated position the vertigo and nystagmus may reoccur in the opposite direction, less violently.
iv. Repositioning or liberatory maneuvers that are shown to be effective include Epley's maneuver, the Brandt–Daroff exercises, and the Semont maneuver.

22 i. Bilateral calcified tumors extending along the optic nerve sheaths consistent with meningiomas, the left extending into the cavernous sinus.
ii. The left third and fourth nerve palsies are due to the presence of meningioma in the cavernous sinus. The bilateral deafness and gait ataxia may be due to bilateral vestibular schwannomas.
iii. NF2. The patient had multiple meningiomas and bilateral vestibular schwannomas. This is characteristic of type 2, or central, NF. The disease is due to a mutation in chromosome 22 of a gene coding for a protein known as Merlin. This is an example of a mutation in a tumor suppressor gene causing multiple tumors.

23

Diary 1

		Time	Pain severity out of 10 (Date:)
Co-proxomol	2.30		
Improvement	3.30	1	
		2	
8 o'clock	8.00	3	
Tablets		4	
Improvement	9.30	5	
		6	
		7	
		8	
2 o'clock	2.00	9	
Tablets		10	
Co-proxomol	3.30	11	
		12	
		13	
8 o'clock	8.00	14	
Tablets		15	
		16	
		17	
		18	
		19	
		20	
		21	
		22	
		23	
		24	

Diary 2

		Time	Pain severity out of 10 (Date:)
Co-proxomol	4.00		
Improvement	5.00	1	
		2	
8 o'clock	8.00	3	
Tablets		4	
		5	
Co-proxomol	11.00	6	
Improvement	1.30	7	
		8	
2 o'clock	2.00	9	
Tablets		10	
		11	
		12	
		13	
8 o'clock	8.00	14	
Tablets		15	
		16	
		17	
		18	
		19	
		20	
		21	
		22	
		23	
		24	

23 This is a headache diary of a patient who gives a history of this pattern of head pain, daily over the last 5 years (**23**).
i. What is the most likely diagnosis?
ii. What does the diary show?
iii. What is the most important part of the management of this patient?

24 A 34-year-old female explains that over the last week or so both legs have felt 'funny', especially when getting into a hot bath when the water feels cooler than she is expecting. In addition, when walking the floor feels rubbery, and she is unsteady if she has to get out of bed in the dark at night. She is also having to pass urine more frequently. In the past, she had an episode where the vision in the left eye was blurry, which took about 3 months to clear up. It was never diagnosed properly, but her GP said it was an attack of 'neuritis' and not to worry about it. On examination, her legs are slightly stiff with brisk reflexes, and there is a sensory level to pinprick to the mid-abdomen. The remainder of the examination is normal.
   What is the diagnosis?

23 i. This patient has chronic daily headache with analgesic overuse.

ii. The diary shows typical analgesic rebound headaches, improved each time with further analgesic intake.

iii. The most important part of the management is to withdraw the analgesics. The current operational definition of daily headache is >15 days of headache each month. Population based 1-year prevalence rates of chronic daily headache are about 4%. At least half of these patients are overusing acute-relief medications. The majority of patients presenting to neurology clinics with chronic daily headache are overusing acute-relief medications. Most give a pre-existing history of a primary headache syndrome, most commonly migraine. The mean duration of primary headache is 20 years, the mean time of admitted frequent medication use at least every second day is 10 years and the mean duration of daily headache is 6 years. It seems that the frequency of acute-relief medication use is more important rather than total consumption. Ergotamine, caffeine, the 'triptans' and almost all types of analgesics alone have been implicated. The latter group includes codeine, paracetamol and aspirin.

Withdrawal of acute-relief medication results in improvement in many but not all patients. The average 'analgesic washout period' before significant improvement is observed is about 3 months. Once acute-relief medication has been withdrawn, prophylactic agents are more effective. Management of these patients should be aimed at minimizing the use of abortive treatment and introducing suitable prophylactic therapy.

24 She currently has an upper motor neuron syndrome to approximately T10. In the past, she had an episode of uniocular visual blurring lasting for 3 months. Whilst there is no evidence of it now clinically, it sounds like optic neuritis. In this situation where there is a new anatomically separate lesion separated in time, the diagnosis is highly likely to be multiple sclerosis, in this case relapsing–remitting. Sometimes the signs of old episodes are absent as in this case, although equally she could have been left with left optic atrophy and a relative afferent pupillary defect. It would be important to rule out a compressive cord abnormality, rendering the previous episode a red herring; alternatively, other multi-focal inflammatory disorders should be considered such as sarcoidosis and lupus.

25 With regard to question 24:
i. What are the cardinal investigations?
ii. What treatment would you give?

26 A 40-year-old female with 10 years of progressive ataxia has the pedigree (26a) and brain MRI (26b) shown.
i. What is the inheritance pattern shown in the pedigree?
ii. What does the MRI show?
iii. What are the diagnostic possibilities?
iv. Is DNA testing available for the differential diagnosis?

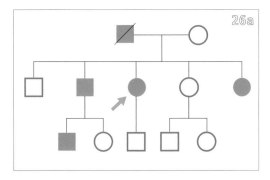

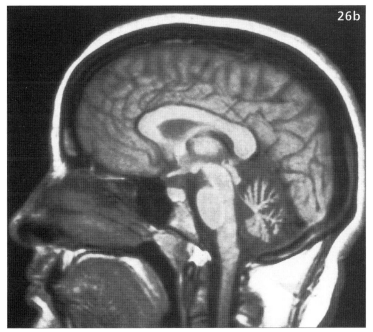

25 i. The essential investigations after a FBC, ESR, B_{12} and folate, autoimmune profile, ACE, and CXR would be MRI brain and cord, VER (searching for the previous lesion), and CSF examination (95% of those with multiple sclerosis will have a pattern of oligoclonal bands that is different and greater than the serum). Her cranial MRI shows characteristic inflammatory demyelinating lesions which are both peri-ventricular and involve the corpus callosum.

ii. Acutely, she is likely to recover by herself. If she worsens then a 3-day course of i.v. methyprednisolone (1 g/day) will hasten her recovery, but probably have no effect on the overall course of the disease. In the long term, if she has two attacks in 2 years and remains ambulant (to more than 100 m) then she would fulfill the current criteria for beta-interferon (Association of British Neurologists). Symptomatic treatment for the future would include anti-spasmodics, e.g. baclofen, and bladder stabilizing agents, e.g. oxybutynin.

26 i. The inheritance pattern shown in the pedigree is autosomal dominant. There is more than one generation affected with male-to-male transmission, ruling out X-linked inheritance and autosomal recessive inheritance. Transmission by a male also eliminates mitochondrial inheritance.

ii. The MRI shows severe midline cerebellar atrophy.

iii. This patient has a hereditary ataxia and most probably has one of the spinocerebellar ataxias (SCAs). The hereditary ataxias are a group of neurogenetic disorders producing slowly progressive incoordination of gait, associated with dysmetria, dysarthria and poor coordination of eye movements. These are slowly progressive and often associated with cerebellar atrophy. The ADCA includes 10 SCAs, SCA1–11 (SCA9 not known), plus DRPLA and two episodic ataxias. Great overlap is present in the clinical manifestations of these SCAs, both in terms of age of onset and physical findings. There are a few distinguishing features for each type. SCA2 shows early slow saccadic eye movements and hyporeflexia. In SCA4 a sensory neuropathy is common. SCA5 has an early-onset ataxia with a slow prolonged course. SCA6 has a later onset of an isolated ataxia with a slow prolonged course. SCA7 often has visual loss with retinopathy. SCA10 presents with ataxia and sometimes seizures. SCA11 is an uncomplicated cerebellar ataxia. DRPLA would be another diagnostic consideration, but is less likely in this patient who does not have seizures, dementia or chorea.

iv. There is highly specific DNA testing available for SCA types 1–3, 6, 7 and for DRPLA. All have trinucleotide expansions in their genes. Tests are not presently clinically available for SCA4, 5, 8, 10, 11.

27 i. What does this picture show (27)?
ii. What are the differential diagnoses?
iii. What investigations would help confirm the diagnosis?

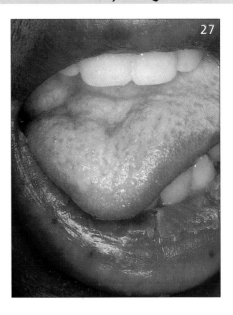

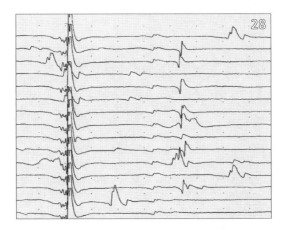

28 A 59-year-old female was admitted with acute urinary retention. She had progressive cognitive decline over the previous 4 years, and had marked gait ataxia and mild cog-wheel rigidity on examination. A CNEMG study was recorded from the external anal sphincter. One MUP from this study is shown in raster display (28).
i. What is the EMG abnormality?
ii. What is the likely diagnosis?
iii. Explain the association between the EMG findings and this condition.

27 i. Wasting of the right side of the tongue with deviation of the protruded tongue to the right.

ii. The differential diagnoses are: (1) A lower motor neuron lesion will cause wasting of the tongue with deviation of the protruded tongue to the same side. The lesion could be in the hypoglossal nucleus (12th cranial nerve nucleus), in the medulla (neuronopathy), or along the course of the 12th cranial nerve from the brainstem, through the hypoglossal canal just below the jugular foramen), to between the jugular vein and carotid artery, forward to supply the muscles of the tongue. (2) Brainstem lesion – tumor, e.g. primary brainstem glioma, metastasis; vascular, e.g. vascular malformation and hemorrhage; asymmetrical syringobulbia. (3) MND – when the tongue is affected in this condition, the wasting is usually more symmetrical than is seen in this patient. Fasciculations are often pronounced. (4) Lesions affecting the 12th cranial nerve: tumors, e.g. malignant meningitis, meningioma, neurofibroma of the 12th cranial nerve; neuropathy which is much rarer, e.g. CIDP; inflammatory diseases, e.g. sarcoidosis; infections, e.g. TB meningitis. (5) Paget's disease – if this affects the skull base, it can cause narrowing of the exit foramina of the cranial nerves, including the hypoglossal nerve.

iii. Investigations that would help confirm the diagnosis are: (1) MRI brain scan. This would provide images of the lower brainstem (CT scanning does not provide adequate images of the brainstem), to enable visualization of space-occupying lesions in and around the brainstem. The use of gadolinium may clarify the causes of intrinsic and extrinsic lesions, and may also provide evidence of meningeal enhancement, not seen on the plain MRI, indicating either malignant or inflammatory meningitis. (2) Skull X-ray/CT scan with bony windows if a lesion involving bone or bony destruction is suspected. (3) Neurophysiology – nerve conduction studies to rule out a generalized or multifocal neuropathic process, e.g. CIDP and needle EMG examination to assess whether there is evidence of widespread chronic partial denervation, such as in motor neuron disease. (4) Lumbar puncture (only if a space occupying lesion has been ruled out) – the constituents of the CSF and CSF cytology may help in the diagnosis of inflammatory and infective conditions and in malignant meningitis.

28 i. The MUP is polyphasic, of increased duration and associated with late potentials. These features indicate significant reinnervation in the external anal sphincter.

ii. This EMG finding, in this clinical context, is consistent with MSA. This condition can present with features of Shy–Drager syndrome, cerebellar ataxia or atypical parkinsonism. EMG evidence of denervation of the external anal sphincter can be helpful in distinguishing atypical parkinsonism from Parkinson's disease.

iii. The anterior horn cells of Onuf's nucleus are selectively lost in MSA. As a result, the striated muscles of the sphincters are denervated.

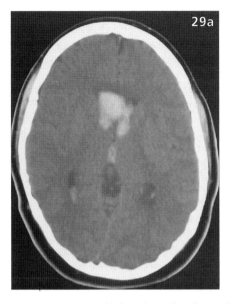

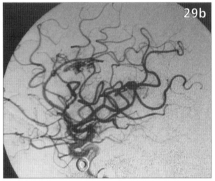

29 This 27-year-old female suffered a sudden onset of severe headache and passed out. Her husband found her and took her to the local emergency department. She regained consciousness in the car and was neurologically intact by the time she was evaluated. A CT scan was performed (29a). Based on the CT scan an angiogram was performed (29b).

i. What does the CT scan demonstrate, what is the leading differential diagnosis, and why was the angiogram performed acutely?

ii. What does the angiogram show, how would you classify this lesion, and what is its natural history?

iii. What are the various treatment options and what are the relative pros and cons to each?

30 During surgery, the patient's end-tidal pCO_2 increases, pO_2 decreases, he becomes tachycardic, and develops metabolic acidosis.

i. What is the diagnosis and what other clinical findings may be found?

ii. What is the disorder's pathophysiology?

iii. What drugs may be associated with the development of this disorder?

iv. How can this be treated?

29 i. The CT scan shows an intraventricular hemorrhage with associated hemorrhage into the corpus callosum, without interhemispheric SAH. In a 27-year-old patient the most likely cause is either an AVM or a pericallosal artery aneurysm. Urgent angiography is required to differentiate these two pathologies (the latter will require urgent surgical or endovascular management to prevent rehemorrhage).

ii. The angiogram demonstrates a small pericallosal AVM fed by several small branches and drained by both a cortical vein into the superior as well as the inferior sagittal sinus. By the Spetzler–Martin grading system this malformation is grade I (<3 cm [<1.2 in] = 1, 3–6 cm [1.2–2.4 in] = 2, >6 cm [>2.4 in] = 3; deep venous drainage = 1, eloquent location = 1), which is important in terms of the operative risk of resection (combined mortality and morbidity: 3% = grade I, 10% = grade II, 20% = grade III, 40% = grade IV, 75% = grade V). Generally speaking, the natural history of an AVM is that it carries risk of bleeding and seizures. Occasionally, they can cause neurologic deficit either through steal (controversial) or direct compression of vital structures usually by a large venous varix. They can also cause intractable head-aches, especially when situated in the occipital lobe and thalamus. The risk of bleeding is often quoted at about 3% per year, with half of all bleeds leading to some residual deficit. The long-term risk of seizures is dependent on location and is difficult to estimate.

iii. Treatment options include embolization followed by surgery or radiosurgery, surgery alone, or radiosurgery alone. Embolization alone is unlikely to cure safely this AVM as total opacification of the nidus including the venous drainage is unlikely to be possible without precipitating further hemorrhage or embolization of particulate matter (namely NBCA glue) into the distal pericallosal. The lesion is appropriate in size for radiosurgery (<3 cm [<1.2 in] in diameter).

30 i. The patient has malignant hyperthermia. The earliest sign is an increase in end-tidal pCO_2 and tachycardia. The body temperature then becomes elevated (may reach 44°C [111°F] at a rate of 1°C [1.8°F] every 5 minutes) and pulmonary edema develops. Later findings include elevated CPK and myoglobin because of rhabomyolosis.

ii. Malignant hyperthermia is a hypermetabolic state in which calcium is released from the muscle sarcoplasmic reticulum.

iii. It can be precipitated by inhalational anesthetics or the use of succinylcholine.

iv. Appropriate treatment includes removal of the offending agent, dantrolene, hyper-ventilation with 100% O_2, cooling, bicarbonate for acidosis, and procainamide for arrhythmias.

31 A 42-year-old male presents with a history of acute back pain followed by the onset of pain in the calf and lateral portion of the foot. He also notices that he has difficulty standing on his toes. The MRI reveals the lesion shown (31).

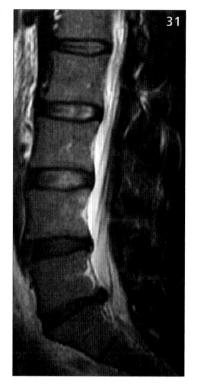

What sign is the most specific for confirming the presumed diagnosis of lumbar disc herniation?
(a) Positive ipsilateral straight leg raise.
(b) Gastrocnemius weakness.
(c) Tibialis anterior weakness.
(d) Absent ankle jerk reflex.
(e) Positive crossed straight leg raise.

32 A 52-year-old healthy, highly successful business executive has been suffering from TGN for 5 years. She has tried several different medications in an attempt to control her facial pain but the paroxysmal attacks have progressed to the point that she often cannot perform her job duties. She has used most of her sick leave and vacation days when her facial pain was too severe, and is at risk of losing her job. Her neurologist has recommended surgical treatment but the patient cannot afford a lengthy convalescent period and prefers not to return for treatment every few months.

What surgical therapy would you recommend?

31 (e). The patient is exhibiting signs of an S1 radiculopathy secondary to a herniated nucleus pulposus at the L5–S1 level. While the straight leg raise test is moderately sensitive in diagnosing a herniated disc (80%), the crossed straight leg raise test is much less sensitive (20–30%) but far more specific (>90%) for confirming the suspected diagnosis.

32 The most appropriate therapy for this particular patient would be treatment at the gasserian ganglion level. The ganglion has three major peripheral divisions, each exiting the skull via a different foramen. The ophthalmic division (V1) exits via the superior orbital fissure, the maxillary division via the foramen rotundum, and the mandibular division (V3) via the foramen ovale. Of the aforementioned foramina, the foramen ovale is the safest and most accessible. The primary treatments commonly used to address the trigeminal ganglion are percutaneous RF ablation, retrogasserian glycerol rhizotomy, and percutaneous balloon microcompression. All of these techniques gain access to the ganglion via the foramen ovale by piercing the cheek (or via an intraoral route) with an 18–20 gauge needle and employing predefined landmarks in choosing a trajectory (32).

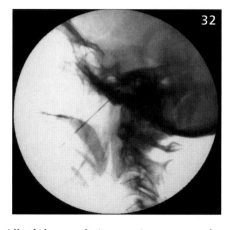

Once access has been gained to the ganglion, various methods are used in the lesioning process. Electrocoagulation, chemical ablation, and physical compression have all been used, each with its own advantages and disadvantages. RF ablation provides immediate relief of pain and has low mortality and recurrence rates. However, it requires specialized equipment and training, may produce corneal anesthesia and keratitis, may produce sensory loss beyond the area of pain, and may rarely produce intractable anesthesia dolorosa (continuous, unrelenting pain which is unresponsive to analgesics and very difficult to manage). These complications are rare, and RF thermocoagulation is the commonest surgical procedure in the management of TGN. Percutaneous retrogasserian glycerol rhizotomy, first described more than two decades ago, is a relatively inexpensive and simple method compared to RF ablation. It has a lower rate of sensory loss, few reports of anesthesia dolorosa, almost no mortality, and is less stressful and quicker to perform. Pain relief however, may take 7–10 days to occur, and the recurrence rate is somewhat higher than with RF ablation. Percutaneous microcompression involves placing a balloon into Meckel's cave and compressing the gasserian ganglion. This technique requires general anesthesia with intubation, and can produce bradycardia and hypotension (as can some of the other techniques) during filling of the balloon. This would make patients with cardiac disease unsuitable candidates. Overall, procedures at the level of the ganglion are the most popular surgical treatments for TGN, and in general, provide upwards of 80% pain relief for at least 3–4 years with minimal morbidity. Gamma knife radiosurgery would be another option for this patient.

33 The following CT scan post-contrast (33) is taken from a lethargic 27-year-old male with AIDS who became progressively stuporous over the course of several hours.

Given the CT scan and the patient's current state, what is the best approach to initial treatment?
(a) Obtain an MRI scan.
(b) Mannitol 100 mg i.v.
(c) Decadron (dexamethasone) 10 mg i.v.
(d) Repeat CT scan in 6 hours.

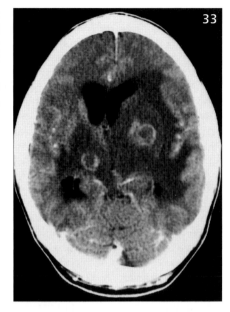

34 This MRI reveals an enhancing mass in a patient with TSC who has suffered an epileptic seizure (34).
i. What is the diagnosis?
ii. What is the appropriate treatment?

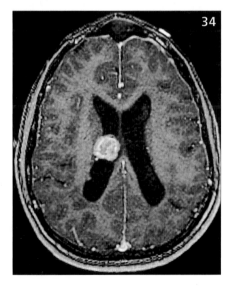

35 i. Describe the major types of functional tumors of the pituitary gland.
ii. Describe the effects of a mass lesion in the pituitary region.

43

33 (c). The contrast CT scan reveals two ring-enhancing lesions with marked cerebral edema, located deep within the brain. Radiographically these areas appear consistent with brain abscesses most likely due to toxoplasmosis. Although most patients with intact mental status can be treated with anti-toxoplasmosis medication, the presence of severe vasogenic edema and depressed level of consciousness warrants immediate treatment with high dose corticosteroids. Mannitol can be given urgently to control *generalized* increased ICP but usually at starting doses of 1 g/kg with the usual initial dose given as 100 g i.v.

34 i. Sub-ependymal giant cell astrocytoma.
ii. The natural history of these lesions is not clear. Surgical excision is generally performed if the lesion is symptomatic.

35 i. The most common functional pituitary tumors secrete ACTH, prolactin, or GH. Other types of pituitary adenomas include those that secrete thyroid stimulating hormone, gonadotrophic hormones (i.e. leutinizing hormone and follicle stimulating hormone), and inactive adenomas that do not secrete any hormone (which overall represent the majority of pituitary tumors) (35). The oversecretion of each of these particular hormones results in distinct clinical syndromes.
ii. Mass effect within the pituitary region can present clinically with general symptoms such as headache, or more specifically with visual field and cranial nerve defects. Upward pressure on the chiasm initially causes a non-congruous superior temporal quadrantanopia that typically progresses to bitemporal hemianopia. Lateral expansion with encroachment of the cavernous sinus can result in III, IV, V1, V2, or VI nerve palsies (i.e. ptosis, facial pain, or diplopia). Rarely, occlusion of the cavernous sinus can occur as well, presenting as proptosis and chemosis.
In some cases the mass effect compromises normal pituitary function resulting in hypothyroidism (i.e. cold intolerance, myxedema), hypoadrenalism (i.e. ortho-static hypotension, easy fatigability), and hypogonad-ism (i.e. amenorrhea, loss of libido, infertility).

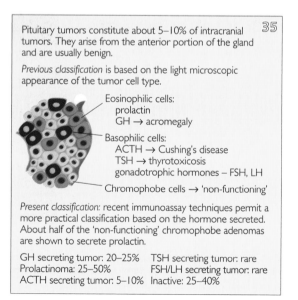

Pituitary tumors constitute about 5–10% of intracranial tumors. They arise from the anterior portion of the gland and are usually benign.

Previous classification is based on the light microscopic appearance of the tumor cell type.

Eosinophilic cells:
prolactin
GH → acromegaly

Basophilic cells:
ACTH → Cushing's disease
TSH → thyrotoxicosis
gonadotrophic hormones – FSH, LH

Chromophobe cells → 'non-functioning'

Present classification: recent immunoassay techniques permit a more practical classification based on the hormone secreted. About half of the 'non-functioning' chromophobe adenomas are shown to secrete prolactin.

GH secreting tumor: 20–25%   TSH secreting tumor: rare
Prolactinoma: 25–50%   FSH/LH secreting tumor: rare
ACTH secreting tumor: 5–10%   Inactive: 25–40%

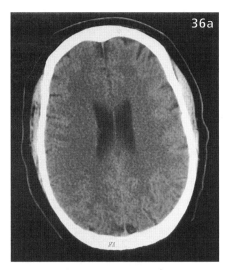

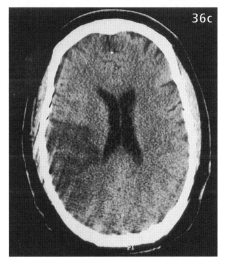

36 A 67-year-old male presents with 6 hours of left upper extremity weakness.
i. What are the findings (**36a–c**)?
ii. What are the early CT findings in cerebral infarct?
iii. What CT findings in acute cerebral infarct contraindicate thrombolytic therapy?

37 A 60-year-old right-handed male complains that for the past 3 years he has suffered from tremor of the left hand. This tremor was first noticed by his wife while he was relaxing watching television. It has deteriorated somewhat and has become a social embarrassment. On examination, he has a slow 5 Hz tremor of the right thumb while at rest and while walking. The tremor is worsened when he is distracted by counting backwards from 100 with his eyes closed. There are no other abnormal findings.
i. What is the diagnosis?
ii. What is the prognosis?

36 i. Nonenhanced (**36a**) and enhanced (**36b**) CT images of the brain at the level of the corona radiata and lateral ventricles show subtle obscuration of the right parietal cortex. A second CT (**36c**) obtained 72 hours later shows a well demarcated, low attenuation lesion involving both cortex and subcortical white matter that is typical of a subacute infarct. This infarct is in the vascular distribution of the parietal branches of the MCA.

ii. Most patients will have normal CT scans in the first several hours after an infarct. Early CT findings, when present, include: (1) increased density in the internal carotid, middle cerebral, or basilar arteries; (2) unilateral loss of definition of the insular cortex, the 'insular ribbon' sign; (3) obscuration of the basal ganglia; and (4) loss of cortical definition in a vascular territory. MRI with diffusion imaging is capable of diagnosing reliably acute infarct within 1 hour of symptom onset, and where available, can confirm clinical suspicion of infarct in the patient with a normal CT scan. Helical CT with images acquired during infusion of contrast material can identify arterial occlusion that may respond to thrombolysis.

iii. Gross cerebral hemorrhage and low attenuation changes involving more than one-third of a cerebral vascular territory are imaging contraindications to treatment with thrombolytic agents.

37 i. Benign tremulous parkinsonism. Parkinson's disease may present with a rest tremor without other features of rigidity and bradykinesia. The tremor may be suppressed with the activity of the body part or even upon concentrating on the resting body part. Thus, unlike psychogenic tremor, it may worsen rather than disappear when distracted. The presentation of tremor (and of parkinsonism in general) is often asymmetric or unilateral, but may spread to the other side as the disease progresses. While tremor may be the sole symptom, there may nevertheless be other subtle signs of parkinsonism that allow a confident clinical diagnosis to be made. These may include a slight asymmetry or fatigability of rapid finger movements, or a unilateral loss of arm swing while walking.

ii. The patient may be reassured that it may in fact be many years before other features of Parkinson's disease develop. The tremor is often more embarrassing than disabling when present in isolation. It may be treated with variable success by anticholinergic drugs such as benzhexol or by levodopa. However, the former may cause tiredness or confusion, especially in the elderly, while the latter invites concern about the development of dyskinetic side effects later in the disease. As a result, many patients remain off medication.

38 A 44-year-old male cab driver complains of increasingly tripping on his left foot over the year. He now has to be careful when getting out of his cab and has fallen over twice. He also has difficulty in 'holding on' to his urine in between fares. Otherwise he feels well. You examine him and find a moderate asymmetrical spastic paraparesis, with some distal reduction in sensation to the ankles. You also rather surprisingly felt that the reflexes in his arms were pathologically brisk.
i. Where is the symptomatic lesion?
ii. What investigations would you perform?
iii. What is his prognosis?

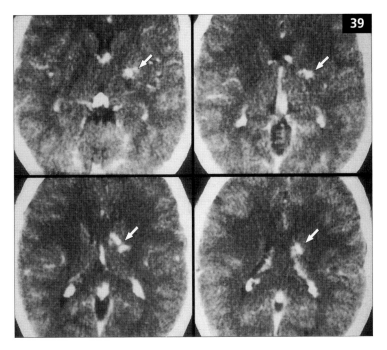

39 A 25-year-old year old male was investigated for a movement disorder. He presented at the age of 21 years with posturing and inversion of his right foot on running. This progressed to involve the right upper limb and he developed writer's cramp. On examination cranial nerves were normal and the only neurologic abnormalities were confined to the right-sided limbs. These showed dystonic posturing and movements of the distal upper and lower right limb. Tone was increased but in a fluctuating manner and power was normal. There was reflex asymmetry with the deep tendon reflexes being brisk on the right. Sensory examination was normal.
i. What does the contrast enhanced CT show (39, arrows)?
ii. How would you investigate and/or treat the abnormality?

38 i. Whilst his legs are affected, on clinical examination his arms are as well, placing the lesion in the cervical spinal cord.

ii. The main investigation would be spinal imaging, specifically cervical MRI to exclude a compressive lesion(s), e.g. spondylopathy. In fact, this revealed atrophy, and cranial imaging demonstrated multiple white matter lesions of increased signal on T_2, making the diagnosis multiple sclerosis. Here there is progressive disease, without the relapsing-remitting pattern classifying the illness as primary progressive multiple sclerosis (PP-MS).

iii. A reasonably large study of 216 patients with PP-MS found a mean age of onset of about 40 years, with a rate of deterioration from onset with was more rapid than relapsing-remitting multiple sclerosis. The median times to reach disability scales of 6 ('intermittent or constant assistance required to walk 100 m') or 8 ('wheelchair bound') were 8 and 18 years respectively.

39 i. The CT scan shows enhancing lesion in the region of the left lentiform nucleus. There are a number of distinct elements to it and the findings would be compatible with that of an AVM. The patient's symptoms were of hemi-dystonia and these findings should alert any clinician to an underlying secondary cause for the dystonia. It is unusual for primary or idiopathic dystonia to present in this way. In adults, dystonia presenting in this way usually suggests a lesion of the basal ganglia including slow growing tumors such as a glioma, AVM or ischemic lesions. In immuno-compromised individuals atypical infections should be considered. Most frequently the lesions affect the putamen.

ii. The AVM should be investigated with formal angiography. This is to identify the extent of the lesion and also any risk factors for subsequent bleeding such as aneurysmal dilation of the vessels or high flow shunts. Neurosurgery for this lesion is a high risk procedure and, depending on the underlying anatomy, the options are endovascular obliteration, radiosurgery or no active treatment.

40 An infant born at 30 weeks was diagnosed with an intraventricular hemorrhage at 23 weeks by *in utero* ultrasound. He has a normal head circumference at birth. Serial head circumference measurements are stable for the first 3 months and then begin to climb over the 95th percentile for his age. Brain MRI (axial T1-weighted image) is shown (40).

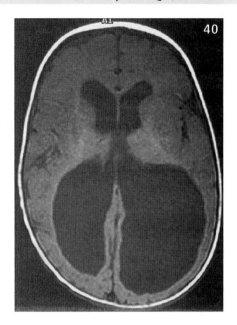

i. What does the MRI show?
ii. Is it likely to be communicating or non-communicating?
iii. What features on the MRI demonstrate elevated ICP?
iv. What clinical symptoms and signs would confirm your diagnosis?
v. What is the best treatment for this patient?

41 A 26-year-old male, unrestrained driver is found unconscious in a roadside ditch. He is intubated and brought to the emergency department with a blood pressure reading of 110/70 mmHg (14.7/9.3 kPa). He is comatose and does not open his eyes to painful stimuli. His pupils are asymmetric: the left pupil is larger and sluggishly reactive. He demonstrates decerebrate posturing to sternal rub.

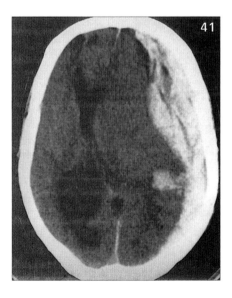

i. How should he be initially managed?
ii. What is his GCS?
iii. Describe the findings on his head CT (41)?
iv. Following his head CT he becomes hypotensive. Is this likely to be due to his head injury?

40 i. The brain MRI demonstrates hydrocephalus.

ii. After an intraventricular hemorrhage, the hydrocephalus is likely to be communicating (non-obstructive) because CSF circulation is blocked at the arachnoid granulations, causing the entire ventricular system to be enlarged. This is in contrast to non-communicating hydrocephalus (obstructive), where CSF circulation is blocked proximal to the arachnoid granulations, causing enlargement of the ventricles only proximal to the blockage.

iii. In addition to enlarged ventricles, the absence of visible cerebral sulci, small sylvian fissures, and a thinned cortical mantle occipitally all suggest increased ICP.

iv. Children with hydrocephalus have macrocephaly with increased head circumference. Additional signs may include bulging fontanelles, splayed cranial sutures, enlarged scalp veins, impaired upgaze, irregular respirations with apneic spells, and bradycardia. Common symptoms are irritability, poor head control, and poor feeding.

v. The best treatment for hydrocephalus in this patient is insertion of a ventriculoperitoneal shunt.

41 i. Following blunt trauma, all patients should be systematically assessed and resuscitated in a standard fashion such as those outlined in the ATLS protocols. Despite obvious neurologic signs, there should be careful assessment for other potentially life-threatening injuries such as ruptured abdominal viscus or bleeding pelvic fracture which may require volume resuscitation. Avoidance of hypotension is critical in preventing secondary neural injury.

ii. The GCS is a means for scoring mental status and assessing change over time of neurologic condition. It is calculated by summing three components: eye opening, best verbal response and best motor response. Because this patient does not open his eyes even with pain (E-1), is intubated (V–T) and shows decerebrate posturing (M–2), his GCS is E1VTM2 = 3T. Coma is indicated by a GCS <8. A GCS of 3T is often associated with a poor outcome.

iii. The head CT demonstrates acute blood layered along the hemisphere with mass effect and midline shift. There is associated parenchymal injury. This is the typical appearance for an acute subdural hematoma, which results from translational acceleration from high velocity mechanisms. Cerebral veins rupture, resulting in bleeding and underlying contusions. The treatment is surgical evacuation when there is significant mass effect, control of intracranial hypertension, and avoidance of secondary insult such as hypotension and hypoxia. Mortality is high.

iv. Hypotension in the acute phase following head injury is rare. It usually indicates systemic injury associated with blood loss. As a rule, increased ICP in isolated head injury is associated with hypertension.

42 A 68-year-old male presented with wasted hands bilaterally (42).
i. Give four causes of this presentation.
ii. What features in the neurologic examination would help to distinguish these causes?
iii. If there were no sensory abnormalities, list four possible causes and the investigation of choice for each.

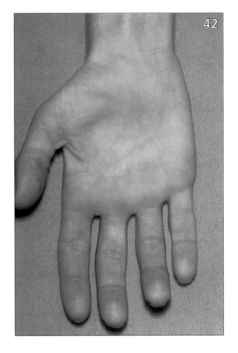

43 A 30-year-old male with a 3-month history of morning headaches, dizziness and facial numbness was noted to have bilateral papilloedema and horizontal nystagmus.
i. What does the MRI scan (43) show?
ii. What is the most likely diagnosis?
iii. What is the prognosis?

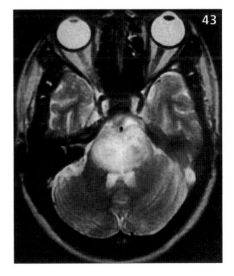

42 i. Wasting of the small hand muscles indicates a lower motor neuron condition. It can be caused by conditions affecting any part of this pathway from the peripheral nerve to the anterior horn cell. (1) Neuropathy (peripheral sensorimotor or motor neuropathy: hereditary, e.g. HMSN; acquired, e.g. CIDP. (2) Bilateral brachial plexopathy. (3) Neuronopathy (i.e. anterior horn cell): MND; ALS. (4) Myelopathy (syringomyelia): a centrally expanding lesion involving the anterior horn cells responsible for the small hand muscles.

ii. The features associated with the wasted hand muscles will help either to localize the lesion or to indicate a possible diagnosis. As well as involvement of the lower motor neuron, as indicated by the wasting of the muscles, additional abnormalities in other parts of the neurologic examination will narrow down the differential diagnosis. Consider abnormalities in the cranial nerve examination, changes in tone, patterns of weakness, the pattern of the reflexes and plantar responses, and the sensory examination: (1) bulbar involvement (MND/syringobulbia); (2) marked fasciculations (MND); (3) spasticity, e.g. MND and in the legs in syringomyelia; (4) pattern of weakeness, e.g. distal in peripheral neuropathy and pattern of particular part of the brachial plexus; (5) reflexes and plantar responses, e.g. it may be brisk in MND with extensor plantars, reduced or absent in neuropathy and plexopathy, and reduced or absent in arms and brisk in legs in syringomyelia; (6) sensory abnormalities, e.g. absent in MND, glove and stocking in peripheral neuropathy, and a cape distribution of pain and temperature loss (spinothalamic tracts) and intact joint and two-point sense (posterior columns) – so-called dissociated sensory loss.

iii. The causes of a pure motor syndrome causing wasting of the small hand muscles are few – either a neuronopathy or a motor neuropathy. In this context, MND is the most likely neuronopathy. The causes of a pure motor neuropathy are also limited and usually one of the following: MMNCB/CIDP, lead neuropathy, or neuropathy secondary to acute intermittent porphyria. The investigations are as follows: for MND, neurophysiology (normal NCS with denervation on needle EMG); for MMNCB, neurophysiology (evidence of conduction block on NCS which may be proximal); for lead poisoning, 24-hour urinary lead; for acute intermittent porphyria, urinary urobilinogen and porphobilinogen.

43 i. Diffuse infiltration and expansion of the brainstem characteristic of an intrinsic tumor. The basilar artery is enveloped by the mass.

ii. Brainstem glioma.

iii. This disease carries a poor prognosis in children with an almost 100% mortality by 2 years. In adults it runs a more indolent course, and in a recent series the median survival was 54 months. Radiotherapy is the only treatment which may be helpful. The radiologic appearances are so characteristic that diagnostic biopsy is usually not warranted.

44 A 35-year-old male with a history of 20 years of progressive ataxia has a normal serum vitamin E level and an abnormal ECG. He has a living 30-year-old sibling in a wheelchair. Their parents are normal.
i. What is the most likely diagnosis?
ii. What are the typical clinical features?
iii. Is there DNA testing available for this disease?

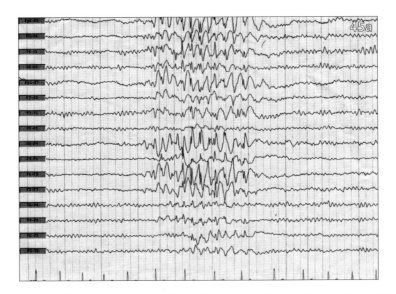

45 A 16-year-old male presents with his first tonic–clonic seizure after missing a night's sleep. His previous medical history was unremarkable, but he had noticed over the preceding 2 years that he would have jerks of either arm soon after waking that could result in him spilling his morning tea. An EEG was performed (**45a**).
i. What does the EEG show, what is the likely diagnosis and what other seizures are associated with this syndrome?
ii. What precipitating factors should he avoid?
iii. What is the treatment of choice, and for how long will he need to be treated?

44 i. The most likely diagnosis is FRDA.
ii. FRDA is characterized by a slowly progressive ataxia of gait and limbs associated with hyporeflexia, extensor plantar responses, loss of position and vibration senses, dysarthria and cardiomyopathy. Its onset is usually before the age of 25 years. Approximately 20–35% of cases may have a later onset (after age 25 years) and have retained deep tendon reflexes. Other frequent signs are glucose intolerance or diabetes, scoliosis, pes cavus, optic atrophy and deafness. It is an autosomal recessive disease. Each child of normal carrier parents is at a 25% risk for inheriting the disease.
iii. There is DNA testing available. The gene is at chromosome 9q13 and the majority of patients with FRDA (~96%) are homozygous for a GAA expansion in intron 1 of this gene. The rest of the patients are heterozygotes for a GAA expansion in one allele and a point mutation in the other allele.

45 i. The EEG shows a generalized epileptiform burst (polyspike and slow-wave) consistent with a generalized epilepsy. The combination of early morning jerks, tonic–clonic seizures and age of onset are typical of JME – one of the idiopathic generalized epilepsies. Absence seizures may also occur. Absences are typically associated with a 3 Hz spike/wave discharge on the EEG (45b). There is often an associated family history of epilepsy.

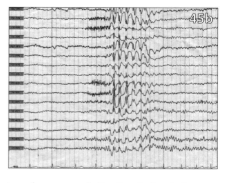

ii. Seizures in idiopathic generalized epilepsies often occur following lack of sleep or alcohol consumption. In addition, photosensitivity is common in JME, occurring in up to 30% of cases. The flicker frequency that usually results in a discharge is 10–25 Hz. Although the flicker frequency of television (50 Hz) is higher, harmonics in this frequency can induce seizures. This risk can be minimized by sitting further from the screen in a well-lit room. Computer screen flicker frequency is much higher and is unlikely to induce a seizure. The content of a game, however, may contain objects that flicker at a frequency liable to induce seizures.
iii. Sodium valproate is the treatment of choice. Carbamazepine and phenytoin can worsen both the myoclonus and the absences. Clonazepam can be helpful for the myoclonus, and there have been reports of the effectiveness of some newer anti-epileptic drugs in this syndrome (especially lamotrigine). Although JME responds well to treatment, most (90%) will need life-long treatment. This contrasts with other epilepsy syndromes in which overall about 60% of those who become seizure-free can expect to come off medication, and other childhood idiopathic generalized epilepsies that usually spontaneously remit in adulthood.

46 A 43-year-old female gave a history of instantaneous severe pain to the back of the head whilst sitting watching television. The pain had become generalized, throbbing in nature and was accompanied by nausea, vomiting, photophobia and neck stiffness. She was seen the following day in the emergency department. Apart from modest neck stiffness the neurologic examination was normal. A CT head scan was subsequently performed (46).

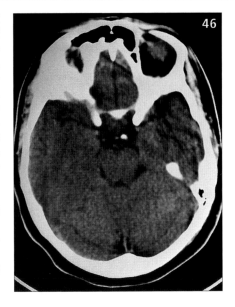

i. What does the CT scan show?
ii. Can a definitive diagnosis be made from this?
iii. What is the next step in the management plan?
iv. What is the prognosis in such a patient with normal initial investigations?

47 The first picture (47a) is of a teased nerve preparation from a sural nerve biopsy of a 50-year-old male who presented with a 2-year history of a relapsing patchy motor and sensory neuropathy. The biopsy was done after nerve conduction studies. The second picture (47b) is an MRI scan of the sacral spine of the same patient.

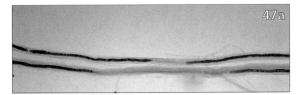

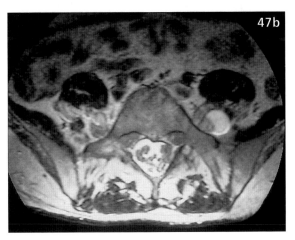

i. What is shown in the first picture?
ii. What does the MRI show and what is the most likely diagnosis from both pictures?

46 i. This patient gives a history of headache with thunderclap onset. The primary concern is to exclude a SAH. The patient has a normal CT head scan.

ii. A CT head scan without contrast performed within 24 hours of onset of the headache can detect aneurysmal SAH in about 95% of patients. This figure drops to about 50% by 1 week and to almost zero by 3 weeks. CT is more reliable than MRI within the first 24 hours, but is inferior to MRI after this time. Therefore a normal CT head scan does not exclude the presence of a SAH.

iii. A lumbar puncture should be performed to look for CSF xanthochromia. Spectrophotometric CSF examination will reveal xanthochromia after SAH in 100% of cases by 12 hours after the initial event. Visual inspection and blood stained CSF are inadequate indicators of SAH. Xanthochromia after SAH is present in 100% of cases from 12 hours up to 2 weeks, in at least 70% of cases into the third week and 40% after 4 weeks.

iv. Headache with thunderclap onset can have a benign course. However, this is a diagnosis of exclusion. A patient with benign thunderclap headache cannot be clinically distinguished from one with thunderclap headache due to an alternative pathology such as SAH. Therefore CT and CSF examination are imperative initial investigations. Long-term follow-up of patients with normal CT and CSF examination suggest a benign course. A small proportion of these patients may subsequently have infrequent recurrence of thunderclap headache whilst almost half give a history of migraine or tension-type headache. Other causes include venous sinus thrombosis.

47 i. This picture (47a) shows two areas of demyelinated segment of nerve with early remyelination.

ii. This MRI shows grossly thickened spinal nerve roots. The combination of a demyelinating neuropathy and grossly thickened spinal nerve roots in this patient suggests the diagnosis is CIDP. CIDP is an acquired demyelinating neuropathy which can present at any age. The neuropathy can be a symmetric motor and sensory neuropathy but more commonly is asymmetric, both clinically and on nerve conduction studies. The neuropathy can be predominantly sensory or motor. MMNCB is generally thought to be a purely motor form of CIDP. The nerve conduction studies in CIDP may show conduction block in some nerves as well as a demyelinating neuropathy. CSF protein is often raised and anti-GM1 antibodies may be present. Nerve biopsy shows demyelination and remyelination, and usually inflammatory cells can be seen in the nerve. CIDP can be seen in association with a serum paraprotein and this should be looked for in all cases. Initial treatment is usually with steroids or i.v. Ig. Ig treatment usually needs to be repeated at regular intervals. Plasma exchange can also be used if Ig treatment is not successful or cannot be tolerated. Further immunosuppression with azathioprine, cyclosporin or cyclophosphamide may be necessary.

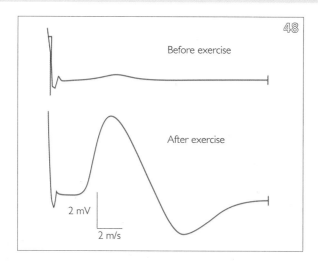

48 A 61-year-old male was referred to the EMG laboratory with a 6-month history of aching in his muscles and difficulty climbing stairs. He also described paresthesias in his feet and had recently begun to notice dryness of his mouth. CMAPs, recorded from the right ADM muscle and elicited by supramaximal stimulation of the left ulnar nerve at the wrist, are shown (48). The top CMAP tracing is from ADM at rest, and the bottom tracing is after maximal voluntary contraction of the muscle for 20 seconds.
i. What abnormalities are evident?
ii. What is the diagnosis?
iii. What other neurophysiologic investigations would be helpful?

49 A 58-year-old male with no significant past medical history has come to seek surgical treatment for his medically refractory TGN. He wishes to undergo a surgical procedure that has the highest success rate, and the longest pain-free interval available. After elaborating on the associated surgical risks of the plethora of available procedures, the patient is adamant in receiving the most effective and long-lasting treatment.
   Which procedure would you recommend?

48 i. The resting CMAP amplitude is markedly reduced. There is evidence of post-activation (i.e. after exercise) potentiation of >200%. This indicates a pre-synaptic neuromuscular transmission disorder.
ii. These findings are indicative of the LEMS.
iii. Repetitive nerve stimulation at slow rates (1–3/s) elicits significant decrement. This is lessened post-activation. Repetitive nerve stimulation at fast rates (>10/s) elicits a marked incremental response, where the calcium ion influx into nerve terminal region induced by the fast stimulus, causes the CMAP amplitude to increase towards normal values. Single fiber EMG can also be carried out, and will reveal increased jitter and blocking.

49 The most effective and longest lasting surgical technique for TGN is micro-vascular decompression, refined and popularized by Peter Jannetta. The procedure is based on the concept that compression of the fifth cranial nerve at the root entry zone by nearby vasculature causes demyelination leading to abnormal electrical conduction and resultant pain. The most frequent vessel causing compression is the SCA (80%), followed by the AICA and basilar artery (**49a**). After performing a suboccipital craniectomy, suspect vessels are mobilized and a small piece of inert material, such as a Teflon pledget, is interposed to prevent compression (**49b**). It is a major neurosurgical procedure but carries <1% mortality, and 3% persistent major morbidity, in experienced hands. Morbidities include intracranial hemorrhage, transient hearing loss, and minor sensory loss. With over an 8-year follow-up period, 60% of patients are pain free and 70% have good pain relief, despite greater than 90% initial pain relief. Microvascular decompression, while associated with a higher mortality and morbidity rate, provides excellent long-lasting pain relief in medically-fit patients suffering from classical TGN. An appealing and viable alternative is gamma knife radiosurgery which provides good to excellent pain relief in 75% of patients, with 75% of responders experiencing good pain relief for a median interval of 18 months.

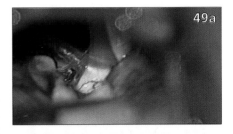

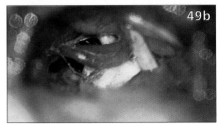

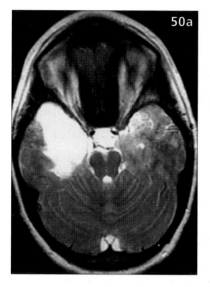

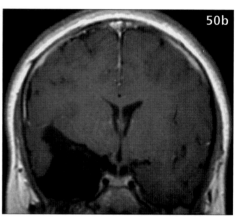

50 A 4-year-old male is referred to your office for evaluation of the lesion shown (50a, b). His parents tell you that they discovered this lesion last year, but elected to follow it because he was asymptomatic. They are now very concerned, however, because he has not been eating well for the past 3 weeks, and that last week he had a seizure for the first time.
i. What is the most likely diagnosis?
ii. What sequence of MRI would be helpful to exclude another type of congenital lesion?
iii. List the indications for treatment of these lesions.
iv. Discuss the treatment options for this patient.

51 A 65-year-old female comes to your office for a check up. She has hypertension and hypercholesterolemia. She is concerned about her risk of stroke and is taking aspirin on a daily basis. She has no history of heart disease and has never had a stroke or experienced an episode of transient cerebral ischemia.
    Will aspirin decrease her risk of stroke?

50 i. The images (**50a, b**) demonstrate an arachnoid cyst. These are congenital lesions that arise during development from splitting of the arachnoid membrane. **ii.** DWI sequences would help distinguish an arachnoid cyst from an epidermoid cyst, another developmental lesion that may arise when retained ectodermal implants are trapped by two fusing ectodermal surfaces. **iii.** Most arachnoid cysts that become symptomatic do so in early childhood. Although the clinical presentation varies with location of the cyst, most children present with symptoms and signs of increased ICP (e.g. headache, poor feeding, lethargy) or seizures. Most neurosurgeons recommend not treating arachnoid cysts that do not cause mass effect or symptoms. Accepted indications for operative intervention include increased symptoms (including

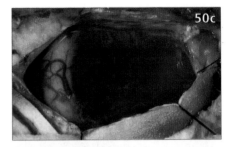

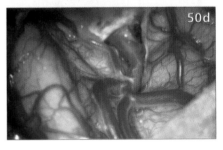

seizure frequency, ICP, or declining neuropsychiatric testing) and increasing mass effect of the lesion. Of note, some authors have advocated earlier operative intervention in these children because of the increased risk of subdural hematomas after even mild head trauma. **iv.** There are three surgical options to treat arachnoid cysts. (1) Drainage of the cyst by needle aspiration is simple and quick, but there is a high rate of cyst recurrence. (2) Craniotomy with excision of the cyst wall and fenestration into the basilar cisterns allows direct visualization to treat effectively any loculations and avoids a permanent shunt in some cases (pre- and post-fenestration shown in **50c, d**). However, a craniotomy has increased morbidity, and subsequent scarring may block fenestration allowing reaccumulation of the cyst. (3) Shunting of the cyst into the peritoneum is definitive treatment with low morbidity and rate of recurrence. The patient becomes shunt dependent, however.

51 Multiple studies fail to support a role for aspirin in the primary prevention of stroke. In fact, most studies show that aspirin increases the risk of ICH when given in a primary prevention setting (i.e. to persons without a prior history of stroke or TIA). Meta-analyses reveal that aspirin is an effective therapy for the primary prevention of MI and likely decreases the risk of ischemic stroke, but the decrease in ischemic stroke is offset by the increase in hemorrhagic stroke. From a public health perspective, aspirin use for the primary prevention of vascular disease is rational since MI is more common than stroke and associated with a higher mortality. In the Physicians' Health Study, where healthy male physicians were randomized to aspirin or placebo, the risk of MI and stroke was greatest among those individuals with the highest C-RP levels, and the benefit of aspirin in reducing cardiovascular disease was restricted to those individuals with the highest concentrations of C-RP. These data suggest that in addition to its anti-platelet activity, aspirin may exert a beneficial effect through its anti-inflammatory activity.

52 With regard to the case in 51, the patient's lipid profile reveals the following: total cholesterol = 6.2 mmol/L (240 mg/dl); LDL = 3.9 mmol/L (150 mg/dl); HDL = 0.9 mmol/L (35 mg/dl).

What intervention is needed for the treatment of her hypercholesterolemia?

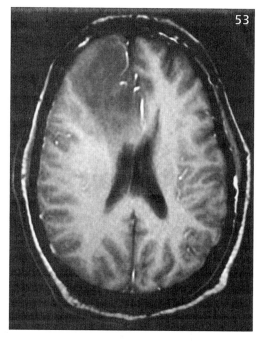

53 A 38-year-old male suffered a generalized seizure. This T1-weighted MR image (53) was obtained after administration of gadolinium DTPA.

i. What are the findings?

ii. What is the most likely diagnosis?

52 The relative significance of cholesterol as a risk factor for stroke has been debated. Epidemiological studies suggest that the risk of ICH is increased in patients with very low cholesterol levels, although the reason for low cholesterol in these patients has never been adequately addressed. The NCEP recommends that the LDL be <3.4 mmol/L (130 mg/dl) in persons with risk factors for cardiovascular disease but no history of heart disease, and <2.6 mmol/L (100 mg/dl) in persons with a history of heart disease. Strict diet can usually effect a 10%–20% decrease in LDL. For persons with significant elevations in LDL, pharmacologic interventions are needed. The only cholesterol lowering agent shown to decrease the risk of stroke is pravastatin, which is an HMG-CoA reductase inhibitor. Whether other HMG-CoA reductase inhibitors, or 'statins', will also prevent strokes is not clear, but it is likely that the benefit will extend to other drugs within the class. The CARE study showed that in persons with heart disease and relatively normal cholesterol levels (average total cholesterol = 5.4 mmol/L [209 mg/dl], average LDL = 3.6 mmol/L [139 mg/dl]), treatment with pravastatin reduced the relative risk of stroke by 31%. The benefits of pravastatin for reduction of vascular disease were more robust in women than in men, and the risk reduction for stroke was seen in older (65–75 years of age) as well as younger patients. The LIPID study was similar in design to CARE and showed a 19% relative risk reduction in stroke in patients taking pravastatin. In both CARE and LIPID, stroke was a pre-defined primary end-point. In a post-hoc analysis of the 4S, a trial of cholesterol lowering with simvastatin in patients with heart disease and elevated cholesterol (average total cholesterol = 6.8 mmol/L [261 mg/dl], average LDL = 4.9 mmol/L [188 mg/dl]), there was also a significant reduction in stroke among patients randomized to statin therapy. Many researchers believe that the benefits of statins are unrelated to their cholesterol lowering properties. Analysis of the patient population from the CARE study showed that pravastatin significantly reduced C-RP levels, and did so independently of its effect on cholesterol. Given the association of vascular events and C-RP levels in the Physician's Health Study, and the fact that aspirin was only beneficial in those individuals with the highest C-RP levels, the benefits of pravastatin in CARE and LIPID are even more remarkable, since most (approximately 81%) patients were also taking aspirin.

53 i. The MRI shows a lesion in the right frontal white matter that extends to the cortex anteriorly and the genu of the corpus callosum posteriorly. The cortical sulci are expanded and effaced. The right lateral ventricle is compressed. The signal intensity is the same as, or slightly lower than that of gray matter, and the lesion does not enhance with gadolinium.
ii. These findings, along with the clinical presentation of a first seizure at age 38 years, suggest a low grade primary glial neoplasm such as astrocytoma, oligodendroglioma, or mixed tumor. While MRI cannot predict accurately the histologic grade of tumor, higher grade neoplasms such as anaplastic astrocytoma or glioblastoma typically demonstrate neovascularity and consequent enhancement. Glioblastoma and metastatic neoplasms often show central necrosis as well, which appears as a low signal intensity lesion surrounded by a high signal, irregular ring.

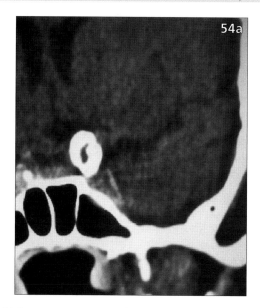

54 This 68-year-old, hypertensive, ex-smoking female presented to her neurologist on referral from her ophthalmologist after he diagnosed her with a partial field cut and decreased acuity on the left. MRA revealed a 1–2 cm (0.4–0.8 in) left paraclinoid aneurysm and a coronal CT scan was obtained as part of a 3D CT scan (54a).
i. Why does the patient have an inferior field cut?
ii. What further testing would you order in this woman?
iii. Would you recommend that she have this aneurysm treated and if so how?

55 A 40-year-old female presents with a long history of unsteadiness on standing. Her first recollection of the problem was when she was taking her marriage vows. She became very anxious and unsteady and started shaking uncontrollably. On sitting down, she rapidly recovered. She has no difficulties with her speech or with coordination of tasks involving her upper limbs. In the last few years, she has also developed unsteadiness while walking. There is no family history, she does not drink and she is on no medications. On examination, she simply finds it impossible to stand for more than a few seconds before grabbing for support or sitting down. Her gait is unsteady and somewhat wide-based. On the examination couch, eye movements, speech, vestibular function and limb motor function, reflexes, coordination and sensation are all normal.
i. What is the clinical diagnosis?
ii. How may this diagnosis be confirmed?
iii. What treatments are available?

54 i. The superior edge of the optic nerve is compressed against the falciform ligament making it ischemic.

ii. As the risk of an angiogram is about 1% given her age and other risk factors, and treatment is unlikely to be recommended at this time, no other testing is necessary. This 1% figure is based on a similar aged population undergoing evaluation for CEA as part of the ACAS trial in the early 1990s.

iii. Given the fact that this aneurysm is in the paraclinoid region, is heavily calcified, and is very minimally symptomatic, the best course of action would be conservative follow-up. This is based on increasing evidence that the natural history of such a lesion is fairly benign with a yearly hemorrhage rate far <1%. Given her life expectancy and the risk of surgery (10% risk of stroke and 10% risk of significant visual deficit), direct surgical reconstruction is not recommended. Although GDC embolization would be significantly less risky for this heavily calcified aneurysm it is unclear whether this therapy does anything to alter the natural history of this disease.

If this aneurysm were to grow on serial imaging, GDC might, at that time, be considered. Endovascular carotid ligation under full heparinization with or without a bypass might also be considered. Unfortunately, direct surgical reconstruction would require an endarterectomy of the neck region which would require considerable cross clamp time and might result in acute carotid occlusion.

55 i. Primary orthostatic tremor. This is a rare condition presenting in middle-age with a rapid leg tremor on standing. Sometimes patients do not perceive the tremor but instead merely report unsteadiness which settles on sitting or walking. Despite being called orthostatic tremor, it is often also manifest on walking, although of lesser severity. On examination, the tremor is generally invisible as it runs at a rapid 16 Hz frequency. Instead, it is better detected as a vibration felt in the postural support muscles.

ii. The diagnosis may be confirmed by electrophysiologic demonstration of polyphasic EMG bursts in postural muscles at around 16 Hz, far faster than the frequency of other tremors. Sometimes subharmonic frequencies at 8 Hz are present, often in the upper limb muscles. This, together with reports of essential tremor in family members of primary orthostatic tremor patients, has led to the belief that the two tremors reflect the same condition. However, the familial associations are probably coincidental, and in essential tremor the oscillatory activity is relatively independent in different limbs, while in primary orthostatic tremor the 16 Hz bursts and even the 8 Hz subharmonics have a fixed timing pattern of EMG bursts in all four limbs.

iii. Primidone, beta-blockers, benzodiazepines (especially clonazepam) and levodopa have all been used to alleviate primary orthostatic tremor with variable success. Clonazepam seems reasonably effective in a significant proportion of patients, while recent reports have indicated that levodopa is beneficial.

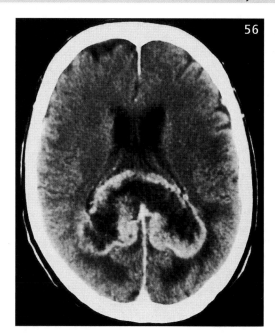

56 i. What is the classic presentation of this condition (56)?
ii. What is the diagnosis and how is it made?
iii. What is the prognosis?

57 A 37-year-old professional diver with a history of classic TGN of 4-years duration hit the back of his head and neck in an accident 2 years prior, luckily without neurologic injury. Approximately 3 months after the accident, he began experiencing chronic progressive stabbing and burning pain on the left side of his occiput. His facial pain is well controlled with carbamazepine and baclofen, but his progressive occipital pain is resistant to medical management and is severely affecting his quality of life.
i. How would you classify the nature of his occipital pain?
ii. What are his current treatment options?

56 i. A short history of dementia and headaches in a middle-aged patient.
ii. Butterfly malignant glioma. The diagnosis is obvious on the contrast CT. Stereo-tactic biopsy would remove all doubt. Resective surgery is not indicated.
iii. Radiotherapy may prolong survival, but the prognosis and future quality of life are poor as the tumor spreads around the splenium of the corpus callosum.

57 i. This patient's occipital pain is an example of peripheral nerve neuropathic pain, also known as occipital neuralgia. It is not uncommon for patients with TGN to concurrently suffer from other types of atypical pain. For example, some patients experience paroxysmal attacks of stabbing facial pain with chronic dull facial pain being ever present in the background. In general, the medical or surgical techniques typically employed in the management of TGN have a good chance of alleviating the paroxysmal pain but tend to unmask the chronic, dull, atypical pain that then becomes the patient's primary complaint. Other patients develop atypical facial pain after classical TGN has been treated surgically as a result of deafferentation. This deafferentation pain has been treated with great difficulty with reassurance, analgesics, tricyclic antidepressants, psychotherapy, and most recently, by chronic epidural facial motor cortex stimulation.
ii. This patient's occipital neuralgia, which has failed medical management, may benefit from other types of surgical treatments. These include nerve blocks, chronic peripheral nerve stimulation, which consists of the placement of subcutaneous electrodes at the base of the occiput overlying the pathway of the greater and lesser occipital nerves (57). After connection to a pulse generator implanted under the clavicle, this device produces unilateral pleasant paresthesias in the area of pain. This modality lessens pain by greater than 50% in approximately two-thirds of patients who otherwise have only few remaining options. For the one-third of patients who fail a trial of peripheral nerve stimulation, an implantable analgesic (typically mor-phine) pump is the next viable option.

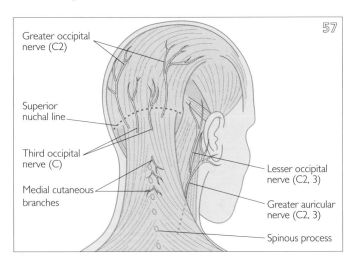

58 On a routine health examination of a 57-year-old female you detect a left carotid bruit and order a carotid ultrasound. The carotid ultrasound suggests that there is ~70% stenosis (58).

Should she undergo endarterectomy?

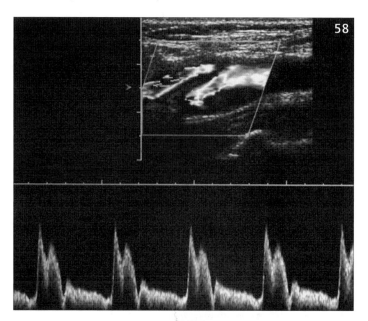

59 Assume, after further history, you discover that the patient in 58 experienced a 5-minute episode of right-sided weakness and language difficulties about 1 month ago. An angiogram is performed and confirms a >70% stenosis (59).

Does this change your recommendation about endarterectomy?

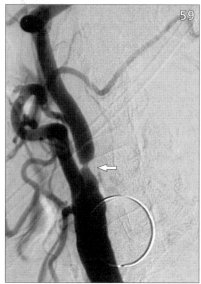

58 Auscultation of a bruit does not necessarily imply the presence of significant carotid disease. Similarly, lack of a bruit does not mean that there is not significant disease. The patient presented above has *asymptomatic* carotid artery stenosis. The ACAS showed that the risk of stroke could be decreased by CEA in patients with ≥60% stenosis of the carotid artery. The 5-year risk of ipsilateral stroke or peri-operative stroke or death was 11.0% in medically treated patients and 5.1% in surgically treated patients, or 2.2% per year and 1.0% per year, respectively. Thus, these data show that surgery decreases the rate of stroke by 1.2% per year. Given the inherent risks of angiography and surgery, however, the benefit of CEA for stroke prevention would not be realized until 1 year after surgery.

There is controversy surrounding the conclusions of ACAS. There was an overall benefit to CEA in the study, but it was small and dependent on very low surgical morbidity and mortality (<3%). In the ECST study, the risk of stroke ipsilateral to an asymptomatic carotid artery stenosis was only 2.1% over 3 years, but increased to 5.7% for persons with severe (70–99%) stenosis. If one could define more accurately the asymptomatic patient population most likely to benefit from CEA, the risk–benefit ratio might better favor surgery. In ACAS, there was no benefit to surgery for women, which may be related, in part, to a higher surgical complication rate among women. The results of ACAS suggest that the population of asymptomatic patients most likely to benefit from CEA is men, especially men with higher degrees of stenosis. Medical management of the person with asymptomatic carotid disease is now well defined, but should probably include aspirin. There is also accumulating evidence that therapy with statins can either slow or reverse the progression of atherosclerotic carotid artery disease.

59 The data for *symptomatic* carotid artery stenosis is less controversial than for asymptomatic carotid artery stenosis. In the NASCET, there was clear benefit to CEA in persons with symptomatic carotid stenosis of at least 70%. The data from several other symptomatic carotid endarterectomy trials, including the ECST, are similar. In NASCET, the 2-year risk of ipsilateral stroke decreased from 26% in medically treated patients to 9% in surgically treated patients, which represents an absolute risk reduction of 17% (or 8.5% per year). The benefits of CEA are not as robust in symptomatic patients with less severe stenosis, and there was no benefit to surgery in patients with stenosis <50%. In patients with carotid stenosis of 50–69%, there was a significant decrease in the 5-year rate of stroke, from 22.2% in medically treated patients to 15.7% in surgically treated patients. For symptomatic patients with moderate stenosis (50–69%), the benefit of CEA was greatest in persons with a recent stroke and in persons with hemispheric symptoms (as opposed to amaurosis fugax). Women with moderate carotid stenosis did not benefit from CEA in the NASCET study.

The role of stenting for carotid artery disease is currently under investigation. While stenting appears to be a promising alternative to CEA, the benefits have not been proven in a prospective randomized trial.

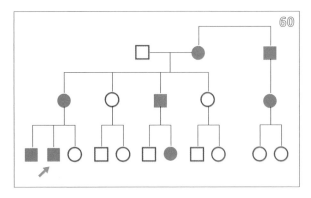

60 An 18-year-old male has bilateral foot drop, distal muscle atrophy, absent tendon reflexes and moderately slow NCVs. His diagnosis is CMT. His pedigree is shown (60).
i. What type of inheritance does the pedigree show?
ii. What type of CMT could he have?
iii. The results of his DNA testing show a mutation in the *connexin 32* gene. What is the diagnosis and what are the risks for CMT to his children if he has a daughter and a son?

61 A 37-year-old nulliparous women presents to the emergency department with a history of a rapid decrease in visual acuity, extreme headache, and decrease in mental status. An imaging study of the patient is shown (61). Upon further questioning of her husband you are told that over the past year the patient has noted significant bilateral discharge from her nipples.

What is the most likely diagnosis and the appropriate course of action/treatment?

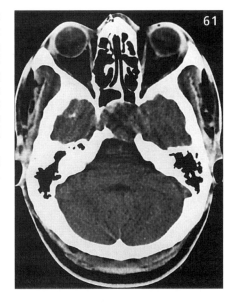

60 i. The pedigree could show either an autosomal dominant or an X-linked inheritance pattern. There is no male-to-male transmission seen in this pedigree which would confirm autosomal dominant transmission and eliminate X-linked transmission. Transmission by a male eliminates mitochondrial inheritance.

ii. He could have CMT1A, CMT1B or CMTX. Charcot–Marie–Tooth disease is the most common genetic cause of neuropathy. It is a group of disorders that produce both motor and sensory neuropathy. There is considerable genetic heterogeneity, that is, many different genes can cause the same phenotype. It can be inherited in an autosomal dominant, autosomal recessive or X-linked manner. The pedigree in this case eliminates autosomal recessive types of CMT. The autosomal dominant form has been divided into two major categories based on the NCVs: CMT1 with slow NCVs and CMT2 with normal or near normal NCVs. CMT1 subtypes A and B are clinically indistinguishable and are designated solely on molecular findings. CMT1B tends to be more disabling and with very slow NCVs, 5–20 m/s. However, some cases of CMT1B are clinically identical to CMT1A. CMT2 has NCVs in the normal, or mildly abnormal range and is unlikely in this case with moderately slow NCVs. Males affected with X-linked CMT (CMTX) have the full syndrome and females may be clinically normal or have mild to moderate signs and symptoms.

iii. The *connexin 32* mutation is seen in CMTX. This means that the patient has X-linked CMT. The risk for his daughters of inheriting the gene is 100%, as he only has one X chromosome, which must have the mutation. For his sons the risk is 0% because they will only inherit his Y chromosome and not his X chromosome.

61 Pituitary apoplexy describes the clinical phenomenon of acute onset of neurologic deterioration due to expansion of a mass within the sella turcica as a result of hemorrhage and/or necrosis. The axial non-contrast head CT clearly shows an area of hyperdensity within the pituitary region consistent with an acute bleed. Given the patient's age and history of galactorrhea it is reasonable to assume that the hyperdensity on CT scan represents hemorrhage from a prolactin secreting macroadenoma. The most appropriate course of action is emergent surgical decompression through a trans-sphenoidal approach.

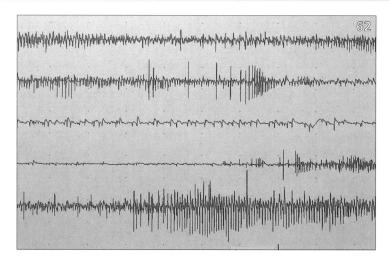

62 A 33-year-old male was referred to the EMG laboratory with a 2-year history of mild weakness in the hands. He and his wife were also attending a fertility clinic. Tracings of the CNEMG study from a resting hand muscle are shown in raster display (**62**).

i. What EMG abnormality is evident?

ii. What is the most likely diagnosis?

iii. Would you expect other EMG abnormalities?

63 A 22-year-old college student was an unrestrained passenger involved in a motor vehicle accident. She was quadriplegic on the scene, but able to breathe without mechanical assistance. Neuroradiologic imaging studies revealed a contusion of the cervico-thoracic cord but no mechanical instability. Over the next few weeks of intensive rehabilitation therapy, the patient slowly regained most of her sensorimotor functions in all four extremities, but a moderate pain/temperature sensory loss persisted. Approximately 7 months following the accident, the patient began to suffer from progressive burning and searing pain in all four extremities with a quality and severity she had never experienced. In addition, she noted increasing weakness in her upper extremities.

i. What would be the next most ideal treatment/diagnostic option?

ii. What are some of the surgical options that may be beneficial in alleviating the patient's symptoms?

62 i. Myotonic discharges occur repeatedly.
ii. The most likely diagnosis is myotonic dystrophy, which is known to be associated with testicular atrophy and infertility.
iii. EMG also revealed low amplitude, short-duration MUPs, many of which were polyphasic in shape. This indicates an additional myopathy, which is of use in distinguishing this condition from other myotonic disorders. EMGs were also abnormal in two of this man's three brothers, and in his mother.

63 i. Pain occurs in approximately 50% of patients with spinal cord injury. In a patient with new and progressive neurologic findings, however, one must always be vigilant for the development of syringomyelia. The next most appropriate diagnostic test in this patient would therefore consist of a cervicothoracic MR scan (**63a** axial and **63b** sagittal T2-weighted sequences) which demonstrates a syrinx (*black arrow*) within the spinal cord (*concave white arrow*), and a normally appearing nerve root (*white arrow*). In patients with stabilization hardware (common after severe spinal column injury) preventing MR imaging, a delayed myelogram CT scan may reveal dilatation of the spinal cord, and/or collection of contrast material within the cord.

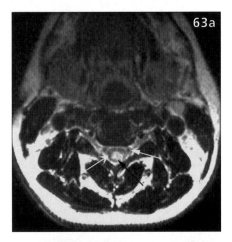

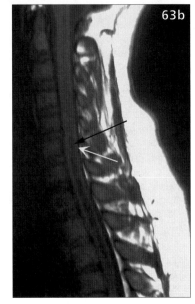

ii. Pain improves in a majority of patients after undergoing shunting of the syrinx, usually via the placement of a syringo-subarachnoid shunt. Additional treatment modalities, including DREZ lesions and medial/ventrolateral thalamic lesions/stimulation, have provided varying degrees of pain relief.

64 A 25-year-old female is referred having had four unprovoked generalized tonic–clonic seizures over the last 6 months She has a mother with epilepsy and she herself is due to be married in a year's time. Examination is unremarkable.

i. What does the MRI show (**64**)?
ii. What other investigations would be appropriate?
iii. What would you advise her?

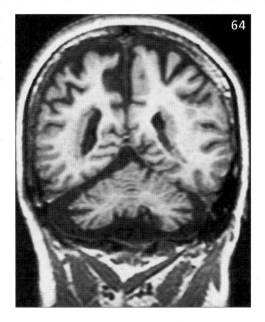

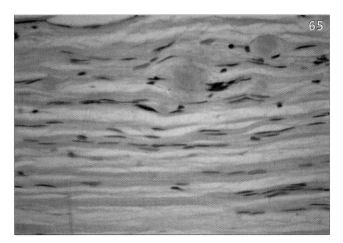

65 A 35-year-old Portuguese male presented with a 2-year history of burning pain in his feet, impotence and postural hypotension. Nerve conduction studies confirmed an axonal neuropathy. A sural nerve biopsy (**65**) was performed.
i. What is shown in this biopsy?
ii. What is the most likely diagnosis?
iii. What treatment should be considered?

64 BPNH. The extensive bilateral heterotopic masses lining the lateral ventricles are of the same signal intensity as cortical gray matter on all sequences. They are not irregular or ovoid, nor are there any cortical lesions. This is not tuberous sclerosis. BPNH is a relatively common developmental cause of epilepsy; seizures may not begin until the second or third decade and, in females at least, cognitive impairment is unusual.

ii. BPNH may be sporadic or familial. Familial cases are most likely to be due to a mutation in the FILAMIN 1 gene (*FLN1*). The gene is on the long arm of the X chromosome. Inheritance is mainly X-linked dominant with male lethality, though the known spectrum of inheritance patterns is broadening. The gene is large (>50 exons) and routine genetic analysis is not widely available. However, the likelihood of a genetic cause could be increased by imaging the patient's mother, who also has epilepsy. If she were found to have BPNH, an *FLN1* mutation is very likely. The patient herself would require baseline hematology and biochemistry prior to consideration of anti-epileptic drug treatment.

iii Three issues need consideration: (1) counseling for epilepsy and prophylaxis with anti-epileptic drugs for the patient; (2) discussion of the issues of contraception, conception, and pregnancy in epilepsy and with anti-epileptic drugs; and (3) genetic counseling.

65 i. The sural nerve biopsy shows areas of homogeneous extracellular material staining red with a Congo Red stain, confirming that the material is amyloid.

ii. The most likely diagnosis in a Portuguese man of this age is TTR FAP due to the methionine 30 mutation in the *TTR* gene. TTR FAP is an autosomal dominant condition originally and most commonly described in Portuguese patients but seen worldwide. In Portuguese patients it usually presents in the third or fourth decade with a predominantly small fiber neuropathy and autonomic involvement. Symptoms due to cardiac and vitreous amyloid deposition are also common. The diagnosis is made by the demonstration of amyloid on a biopsy (usually nerve or rectum). Immunohistochemical staining of the amyloid is used to differentiate TTR from light chain, which is the constituent protein in the more common form of amyloidosis, primary light chain amyloidosis. A valine to methionine substitution at position 30 of the *TTR* gene is a causative mutation in Portuguese patients and can be shown by sequencing the *TTR* gene or by the use of PCR and restriction enzyme digestion. Without treatment, death usually occurs within 10 years due to a severe neuropathy and cardiac complications.

iii. Liver transplantation should be considered. This was first performed for TTR FAP in 1990 based on the rationale that 85% of TTR is produced in the liver. The biochemical effect of transplantation is good with almost complete disappearance of abnormal TTR from the plasma post-transplantation. Operative mortality is about 20% mainly due to the autonomic complications. Although liver transplantation has only been in use for 10 years, it does seem to halt the progression of FAP but the timing is very important. It should be considered early in the course of the disease as duration is the most important prognostic factor for outcome (the longer the disease pre-operatively the worse the outcome).

66 A 5-year-old male with a history of mental retardation and generalized tonic–clonic seizures develops ataxia and a change in his seizure pattern despite stable medications. This prompts the brain MRI shown (66a–c). On physical examination, you notice numerous yellow-brown lesions in a malar distribution.

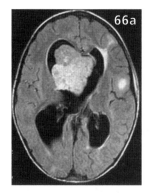
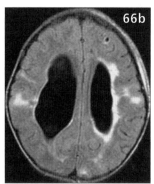
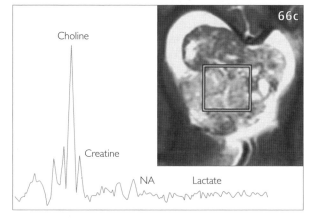

i. What is the most likely diagnosis of the lesion shown on the MRI?
ii. How would MR spectroscopy assist with diagnosis?
iii. What syndrome does this patient have?
iv. How should this lesion be managed?

67 A healthy 70-year-old male complains of difficulty walking, intermittent incontinence, and poor memory that has slowly progressed over the past 2 years. A complete metabolic work-up for dementia is negative, and he is told he has AD. His family tells you that after many months of struggling with his care at home, they have recently decided to place him in a nursing home. Before agreeing with the family, you order a head CT (67).

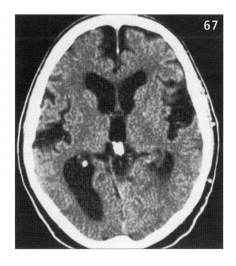

i. What does the head CT show?
ii. Is there an alternative diagnosis?
iii. Can you help this patient?

66 i. MRI scan **66a** shows a giant cell astrocytoma, an enhancing lesion almost always located at the foramen of Monro. They occur in 10–25% of patients with TSC. Imaging studies of patients with TSC also commonly show subependymal nodules, or tubers (**66b**), low density parenchymal lesions representing heterotopic tissue or defective myelination, and hydrocephalus.

ii. Spectroscopy patterns can be helpful to confirm the diagnosis of giant cell astrocytomas (**66c**). Low grade astrocytomas typically have a low creatine to Ch ratio and a low NA to Ch ratio, with an undetectable lactate peak. More malignant tumors tend to have even lower creatine to Ch ratios and NA to Ch ratios, and they develop clear lactate peaks.

iii. The clinical triad of seizures, mental retardation, and sebaceous adenomas are the hallmark for TSC. A neurocutaneous disorder characterized by hamartomas of many organs including the skin, brain, eyes, and kidneys, TSC has an autosomal dominant inheritance pattern, with the responsible gene located on chromosome 9. Additional associated findings include ash leaf macules and depigmented iris.

iv. This symptomatic lesion should be surgically resected. If asymptomatic, paraventricular lesions should be followed closely.

67 i. The head CT demonstrates modest hydrocephalus with enlargement of the lateral and third ventricles.

ii. A likely diagnosis for this 70-year-old man based on the clinical triad of gait disturbance, dementia, and urinary incontinence is NPH.

iii. Yes. Many patients with NPH respond very well to a ventriculo-peritoneal shunt with an improvement in incontinence, then gait, and lastly dementia. Unfortunately, there is no test or radiographic study that is pathognomonic for NPH. Patients who clinically improve after serial lumbar punctures or lumbar drainage are likely to benefit from a ventriculo-peritoneal shunt. To avoid the high complication rates of shunting (nearly 35%) in these elderly patients with fragile brains (e.g. subdural hematoma), many neurosurgeons use programmable valves that allow the shunt pressure to be adjusted from 3 cmH$_2$O to 20 cmH$_2$O via an external magnetic programmer.

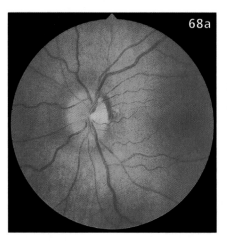
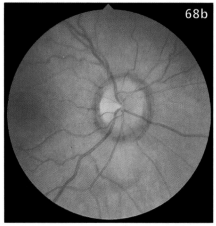

68 A 21-year-old female gave a history of attacks of severe bilateral throbbing headache since the age of 15 years, accompanied by nausea and photophobia occurring once every 2 months. The attacks had generally lasted 1–2 days at a time and she had on several occasions experienced visual aura of 'flickering lights' for 20 minutes prior to the onset of headache. Over the last 3 years the frequency had gradually increased such that she had suffered a mild featureless daily headache for 18 months with more severe exacerbations as described 2–3 times a month. She continued to experience occasional episodes of visual aura, and intermittently over the last few months had complained of blurring of vision. Her current medication was paracetamol as required, and pizotifen 3 mg daily which had improved her symptoms in the past, but less significantly over the previous 6 months.
i. What two main differential diagnoses does the history suggest?
ii. Does the fundoscopic examination (68a, b) further the differentiation?
iii. What are the four first steps which should be taken in the management of the patient?

69 During a craniotomy the patient's end-tidal CO_2 significantly decreases.
i. What is the diagnosis?
ii. What other cardiopulmonary abnormalities may be observed during this event?
iii. When is it most likely to occur?
iv. How can it be detected and treated?

68 i. The patient gives a 6-year history of migraine on occasions accompanied by aura symptoms. The current main diagnoses are of chronic daily headache associated with analgesic overuse and of IIH. The two diagnoses may coexist.

ii. The fundoscopic examination shows papilloedema. The diagnosis can be confirmed by fluorescein angiography which shows diffuse leakage of fluorescein from the dilated superficial capillaries.

iii. Both the paracetamol and pizotifen should be stopped. An MRI head scan should be performed and if there is no evidence of an intracranial mass causing raised ICP, nor of venous sinus thrombosis, a lumbar puncture should be performed. Neuro-imaging is usually normal, although an empty sella or dilated optic nerve sheath on CT may be seen. IIH is confirmed by normal CSF composition (low CSF protein may be present) and raised CSF pressure. The diagnosis is dependent on finding no other cause of raised CSF pressure.

The patient had been taking at least 2 g paracetamol daily for the last 2 years. In view of the association between analgesic overuse and daily headache all analgesics should be stopped. At least 90% of patients with IIH present with headache; three-quarters of this group have daily headache. IIH can cause an exacerbation of headache in individuals who suffer from migraine.

The patient is a young female who is overweight and had gained 10 kg (22.2 lb) whilst taking pizotifen over the last year. IIH is most common in women between 20–50 years and who are obese, or have recently gained weight. The annual incidence rate is 1–2 cases per 100,000 persons, and 19–21/100,000 in obese women aged 20–44 years. The management is aimed at preventing blindness, which can occur in 10% of individuals, and symptomatic treatment for the headache. This includes weight reduction, the use of acetazolamide, loop diuretics, a course of high dose corticosteroids and serial lumbar punctures. In cases of failed medical treatment lumbo-peritoneal and ventriculo-peritoneal shunting have been largely replaced by optic nerve fenestration.

69 i. End-tidal CO_2 decreases with significant venous air embolus.

ii. Other cardiopulmonary abnormalities observed during venous air embolus include: ventilation-perfusion, mismatch, increase in pulmonary artery pressure, decrease in cardiac output, and increase in pulmonary vascular resistance.

iii. Venous air embolus is more frequently seen when a major venous sinus is opened during surgery, particularly when the patient is in a sitting position.

iv. The most sensitive marker of venous air embolism is a precordial doppler. When venous air embolus occurs the wound should be lowered to <30° from horizontal and the patient rotated left side down. Jugular venous pressure can be applied and, if a CVP catheter has been inserted, air aspirated through it. PEEP is ineffective in treating venous air embolus.

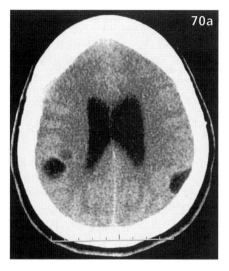
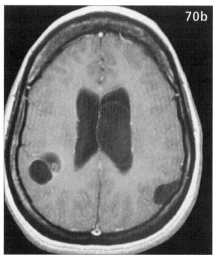

70 A 39-year-old Honduran female with a long history of mild, chronic headaches presents with a generalized tonic-clonic seizure. Neurologic examination was normal. Nonenhanced CT (70a), T1-post-gadolinium MRI (70b) and FLAIR MRI (70c) were obtained.
i. What are the findings?
ii. What is the likely diagnosis?

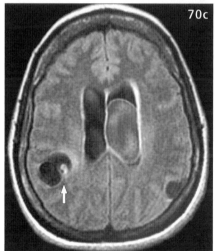

71 Describe how the following anesthetic agents affect the cerebral vascular system and cerebral metabolism, and what side effects they may have:
i. Thiopental.
ii. Ketamine.
iii. Volatile anesthetic agents such as halothane, isoflurane, and enflurane.
iv. Etomidate.
v. Narcotics such as morphine or fentanyl.

70 i. The CT (**70a**) shows enlarged lateral ventricles and several intraparenchymal and subarachnoid cysts without surrounding edema. The MR images (**70b, c**) show an intraventricular thin-walled cyst, two parenchymal cysts at the right parietal gray–white junction, and a left parietal subarachnoid cyst. One of the parietal cysts contains an enhancing serpiginous nodule (arrow).

ii. The constellation of intraparenchymal, intraventricular, and subarachnoid thin-walled cysts in a Central American patient presenting with seizure indicates CNS cysticercosis in its vesicular form. The visualization of an enhancing intracyst nodule is diagnostic of the cysticercotic scolex in this setting. Infection of the CNS by the larval stage of the pork tapeworm, *Taenia solium*, results in formation of intraventricular, intraparenchymal and subarachnoid cysts. The living organism is protected from the immune system and is often asymptomatic for long periods (vesicular stage). When the larva dies, an inflammatory reaction ensues and seizures or focal neurologic symptoms can occur. At this stage (vesiculo-nodular), peripheral edema and ring-enhancement are commonly seen on CT and MRI. Involuting cysts may show enhancement without edema (granular nodular stage). Involuted cysts eventually calcify (nodular calcified stage). FLAIR images are particularly helpful in demonstrating intraventricular cysts, since intraventricular CSF signal is suppressed whilst proteinaceous fluid remains bright.

71 i. Thiopental is a cerebral vasoconstrictor that decreases CBF and $CMRO_2$ but produces cardiovascular depression. Thiopental can protect the brain against the metabolic effects of cerebral ischemia and can reduce ICP.

ii. Ketamine is a dissociative anesthetic that is a pronounced cerebral vasodilator. It increases CBF and $CMRO_2$ during normocapnia. The vasodilatation results in an increase in ICP. Ketamine can also induce seizure discharges.

iii. Halothane is a cerebral vasodilator and increases CBF. When given to patients with even mild intracranial hypertension it causes a further increase in ICP. It decreases $CMRO_2$, however. Isoflurane and enflurane both cause a depression in cerebral metabolism that is associated with cerebral vasodilatation. Among volatile anesthetic agents, isoflurane causes the least increase in CBF. Enflurane can produce seizures. Hypotension and loss of cerebral autoregulation results when the inspired concentration of halothane, isoflurane or enflurane is increased.

iv. Etomidate decreases CBF and $CMRO_2$ but suppresses the adrenocortical response to stress.

v. Morphine in incremental doses causes a progressive and parallel decrease in $CMRO_2$ and CBF. Morphine is a cerebral vasoconstrictor; this effect is abolished by hypercapnic vasodilatation. During normocapnia a combination of morphine and nitrous oxide does not significantly affect CBF or cerebral autoregulation in humans. Fentanyl in normal humans does not have a significant influence on either CBF or $CMRO_2$ under normocapnia.

72 Which test is most sensitive for diagnosing an early post-operative lumber discitis?
(a) Plain radiographs.
(b) Radionuclide scan.
(c) MRI.
(d) CT.

73 A 56-year-old healthy male had a rash in the right V1 dermatomal distribution accompanied by painful vesicular eruptions (73). The rash and vesicles have subsided 4 months ago but unfortunately nagging, burning, and tender pain has developed over the same distribution.
i. How would you label this pain syndrome?

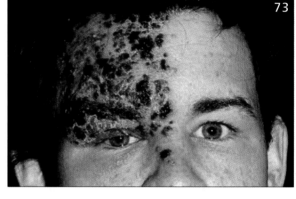

ii. Is there any way of preventing this type of pain from occurring?
iii. What are some of the medical and surgical therapies available in the management of this illness?

74 This 41-year-old female presents with grade I SAH and this aneurysm on cerebral angiography (74).
i. Where is it?
ii. What special surgical procedure helps approach this?
iii. What deficit might you expect post-operatively and how would you manage it?

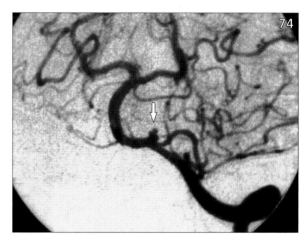

81

72 (c). MRI will indicate low T1-weighted signal and higher T2-weighted signal in the disc space and adjacent vertebral body with a discitis. Plain films and CT rely on destruction of bony structures, which occurs later in the course of discitis. Prior to MRI, the diagnosis was made with gallium or technetium scans but these also rely on structures to become inflamed and take up the isotope. In the relatively avascular disc space and endplate, the early inflammation of discitis will not be found on radio-nuclide scans.

73 i. This patient's facial pain is also known as PHN, and is a consequence of herpes zoster which, in turn, is caused by re-activation of the varicella-zoster virus usually contracted in childhood. With declining immune surveillance accompanying advancing age, or because of an immunocompromised state, the long-dormant virus residing in the trigeminal, geniculate, or dorsal root sensory ganglia re-erupts causing a hemorrhagic inflammatory reaction and re-infecting segmental skin/mucous membrane areas. While pain is usually present before, during, and after the appearance of the rash, the persistence of pain for >1 month once the rash has healed is classified as PHN. Frequently, even long-standing pain spontaneously subsides with time, and only 3% of patients continue to have severe pain 12 months after the rash. The incidence of PHN is directly related to age. While the most common affected dermatomes are in the mid-thoracic region, there is a predilection in the face for the ophthalmic division of the trigeminal nerve.
ii. Systemic steroids have been shown to exert a preventative effect when employed in the treatment of herpes zoster in the immunocompetent patient. Amantadine is an option in patients with a contraindication to steroids, such as those with diabetes mellitus, peptic ulcer disease, or those who are immunocompromised.
iii. For established PHN, low dose amitriptyline, along with a phenothiazine such as fluphenazine, is often an effective form of medical management. Topical capsaicin, the pungent principal of hot paprika or chilli peppers, can be effective, especially if patients can tolerate its side effects (burning after application) for the >3 weeks of daily therapy which is usually required. If medical therapy has failed, surgical lesioning of the dorsal root entry zone is effective for 50–70% of patients. Epidural facial motor cortex stimulation has recently been shown to be an effective alternative in the treatment of this debilitating malady.

74 i. PICA origin.
ii. Far lateral suboccipital craniotomy gives you early control of the vertebral artery and a flatter view across the anterior brainstem.
iii. Lower cranial nerve palsies are usually temporary but swallowing evaluation is necessary before allowing the patient to eat. GDC treated cases often have the same problems (therefore this is an effect of the bleed) and PEG is often necessary.

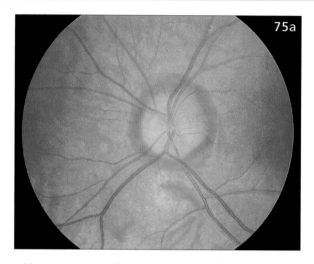

75 A 17-year-old asymptomatic female was referred urgently by her optician for assessment of swollen optic discs (75a).
i. What is the likely diagnosis?
ii. How can this be confirmed?

76 A 42-year-old homosexual male presents with a 6-week history of progressive weakness of the right arm and a 2-week history of language disturbance. On examination, he is apyrexial and general examination is normal apart from some white mucosal lesions intraorally. Neurologic examination reveals a mild expressive dysphasia and a flaccid right arm with MRC grade 3 power proximally and grade 2 distally.
i. What blood tests should be performed?
ii. What is the differential diagnosis of the lesions on MRI (76)?
iii. What other investigations may be performed to confirm the diagnosis?

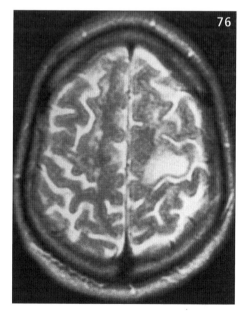

75 i. The likely diagnosis is pseudopapilloedema, with or without buried optic nerve head drusen. The optic disc is elevated, but without any hemorrhages or cotton-wool spots. Also there are no symptoms to suggest raised ICP.

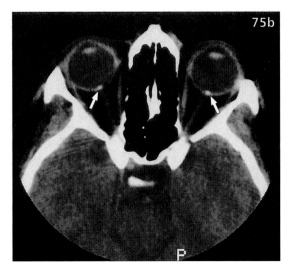

ii. Fluorescein angiography will show no leakage of fluorescein from the optic disc. Buried optic nerve head drusen can be identified as high signal lesions on orbital thin-slice CT scans (75b, arrows) or by ultrasound. Once optic nerve head drusen become exposed, they can be identified by their characteristic autofluorescence.

76 i. The white mucosal lesions could be candidiasis which is usually found in patients who are on corticosteroids (oral or inhaled), diabetics, or patients who are immunosuppressed for any reason such as infection with the HIV. An HIV blood test should be performed and if that is positive then a CD4 count and a viral load should be measured in order to obtain an idea about the degree of immunosuppression.

ii. The differential diagnosis of such lesions in an HIV infected person includes PML, CMV encephalitis and HIV encephalopathy. The symptomatic lesion shown on MRI does not show mass effect or enhancement with contrast and therefore is unlikely to be due to toxoplasmosis or primary CNS lymphoma. CMV encephalitis usually presents more acutely; patients usually have evidence of CMV disease elsewhere such as a CMV retinitis, and MRI may show a periventriculitis. HIV encephalopathy presents with a subcortical dementia but no focal neurologic signs. MRI shows changes that are much more diffuse.

iii. The diagnosis of PML may be confirmed by the detection of the JC virus using PCR. This has a sensitivity of around 80% and a specificity of 95%. A brain biopsy, as performed in this patient, will show the characteristic features of demyelination in association with inclusion bodies within deformed oligodendrocytes and bizarre looking astrocytes.

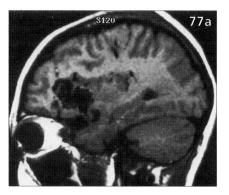

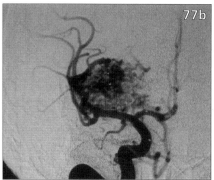

77 This 26-year-old female presented with 10 years of right-sided proptosis and increasing headaches. MRI revealed a lesion (77a). As a result she was sent for an angiogram (77b) which shows this right frontal AVM.
i. How likely is treatment of the AVM to cure or significantly improve her symptoms?
ii. Would you consider this lesion for radiosurgery?
iii. If you were to recommend surgery, would you embolize the AVM pre-operatively?
iv. What surgical approach would you use?

78 A 55-year-old female presents with 18 months of progressive difficulty remembering the names of objects. Although a keen gardener, she finds that producing the specific names for plants is increasingly difficult; for instance, whereas once she would have used words such as daffodil, rose, or tulip she now tends to use the word 'flower' for all. Her husband states that her personal-

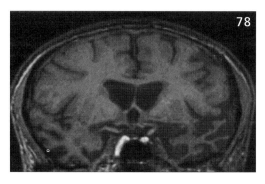

ity has changed over this time, in that she has become obsessed with cleaning the house and she has developed a preference for sweet foods. A formal neuro-psychological assessment confirms that she has difficulty naming objects. It is also noted in the report that she has difficulty on a reading task with words not spelt as they are pronounced (for instance she reads 'aisle' as 'ay-sel' and 'debt' as 'debet'). In contrast, visuospatial ability, such as copying complex figures, is well preserved. Her T1-weighted coronal MRI scan is shown (78).
i. What abnormality is shown on the scan?
ii. What is the clinical diagnosis?
iii. What is the name of this patient's reading disorder?

77 i. The proptosis is related to venous engorgement in the orbit (**77a**). As the shunt is taken down either endovascularly or via surgery this is likely to resolve. The headaches are probably due to stretching of the retro-orbital dura by the markedly enlarged venous varices and should also improve.

ii. This lesion has not bled and is in non-eloquent cortex. A very aggressive radio-surgical dose could be given and if the lesion did not thrombose by 3 years the lesion could certainly be re-treated. However, the true volume of this AVM is really just over 10 ml making cure somewhat unlikely. Embolization and surgery would be reasonable alternative options.

iii. Embolization has the advantage of decreasing the high flow through this malformation, thereby reducing the risk of post-resection perfusion pressure break-through. This phenomenon, felt to be due to shunting of blood into surrounding brain with disturbed autregulatory capacity, is less common since the advent of staged NBCA embolization. Pre-operative embolization also renders the malformation more manipulable which will be helpful in mobilizing the malformation from its attachments along the sylvian fissure.

iv. A pterional craniotomy would suffice here. The sylvian fissure would then be split and the posterior lateral aspect of the malformation followed to the frontal horn of the ventricle. The malformation would then be mobilized from medial to lateral and the subfrontal feeders taken off the ACA. This would leave the malformation pedicled on the large lateral draining vein as it enters the sylvian fissure. This would be taken last. Usually, it is not necessary to divide the sylvian feeders directly off the MCA branches; instead these can be taken subpially in the frontal lobe, lessening the heat transfer onto the important en-passage vessels.

78 i. Focal atrophy of the left temporal lobe.

ii. Semantic dementia (also referred to sometimes as progressive fluent aphasia). This is part of the spectrum of frontotemporal dementia, formerly Pick's disease. As the name implies, patients develop a progressive impairment of semantic knowledge such as for meanings of words and knowledge of objects.

iii. Surface dyslexia. One can only pronounce an irregular word such as debt if one has knowledge of the word. If this knowledge is lost then one can only read according to the rules of phonology, and therefore pronounce the word as it is spelled, in other words according to its 'surface' structure.

79 You are called to the bedside of a patient who has just undergone trans-sphenoidal surgery for resection of a pituitary adenoma. The nurse is concerned because the patient has put out 500 ml of urine in the past 2 hours.

What other information do you need to plan the most appropriate course of action for managing this patient?

80 A 43-year-old male with a history of alcohol use presented to the emergency department initially awake, but rapidly progressed to coma. He was observed not to be moving his left side before becoming comatose. The CT scan (**80**) was obtained.

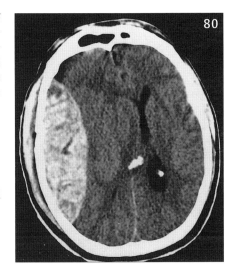

i. What is the lesion seen on CT?
(a) Subdural hematoma.
(b) Subdural hygroma.
(c) Extradural abscess.
(d) Extradural hematoma.
ii. What is the best course of initial therapy?
(a) Obtain an MRI scan.
(b) Urgent neurosurgical consultation.
(c) Decadron (dexamethasone) 10 mg i.v.
(d) Lumbar puncture.

81 A female was accidentally struck in the head on the right side with a golf club. She suffered a momentary loss of consciousness and was noted to have scalp bleeding from the right frontal region, and was brought by her husband to the emergency department awake and alert.

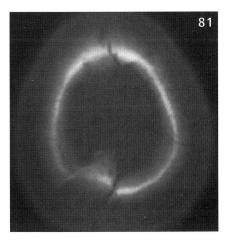

i. Describe her head CT scan (**81**).
ii. What are the important considerations with respect to her injury?
iii. What type of treatment is indicated?

79–81: Answers

79 There are three recognized patterns of post-operative DI that can be caused by damage to the posterior lobe of the pituitary or stalk during trans-sphenoidal decompression. The majority of patients experience transient DI which lasts 12–36 hours post-operatively, characterized by supra-normal urine output and polydipsia. A minority of patients experience prolonged DI which can last months or permanently in up to one-third of this group. A triphasic pattern of DI is observed in an even smaller percentage of patients: characterized first by DI, followed by normalization or SIADH, and finally DI which can be either transient or

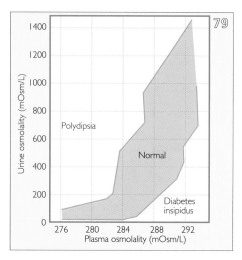

permanent. Other laboratory information helpful in making the diagnosis of DI includes Na+ level and urine specific gravity (79). For patients who can tolerate p.o. intake the optimal treatment for DI is to encourage the patient to drink water. However, when UO exceeds the amount that can be comfortably replaced with p.o. or i.v. fluids (i.e. >300 ml/4 hours), then a vasopressin preparation is appropriate treatment.

80 i. (d) Epidural hematoma.
ii. (b) Emergent neurosurgical consultation. The appearance of the typical lens-shaped lesion on CT represents a large right-sided epidural hematoma. Epidural bleeds are distinctive from subdural blood collections in that they do not cross suture lines and are of arterial rather than venous origin. The result is a rapidly expanding intracranial mass, usually from rupture of the middle meningeal artery, compressing nearby structures leading to overall shift of brain contents and coma. This condition nearly always represents a neurosurgical emergency necessitating immediate evacuation. If evacuated promptly, there can be a rapid improvement in the level of consciousness.

81 i. The head CT demonstrates a skull fracture which is depressed. Because there is an overlying scalp laceration this fracture is classified as an open-depressed skull fracture.
ii. Depressed fractures often lacerate the dura. When they are open the chance of brain infection is significantly increased. When bone fragments are depressed greater than the thickness of the skull, they may be associated with an underlying contusion or hemorrhage. This may lead to an increased risk of seizures.
iii. The proper treatment for this injury is craniotomy for elevation of the depressed skull fracture, irrigation and debridement of the brain and soft tissue injury and dural repair. A short course of antibiotics and seizure prophylaxis may also be warranted. Minimally depressed skull fractures without overlying laceration are usually treated conservatively unless associated with an obvious cosmetic defect.

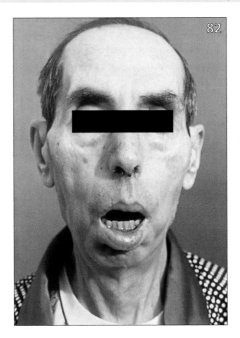

82 This person presents with slowly progressive proximal and distal muscle weakness and difficulty letting go of objects (**82**).
i. What is the most likely diagnosis?
ii. What is the best way to confirm the diagnosis?
iii. What type of potential systemic complications should routinely be anticipated?

83 A 75-year-old male presents with a 2-year history of slowness of gait and small and illegible handwriting. A diagnosis of idiopathic Parkinson's disease is made and levodopa treatment commenced with significant improvement. After another 5 years, following numerous adjustments of his medication, he develops uncontrollable gyrating movements of his arms and legs for about half an hour after taking each of his five doses of Sinemet-Plus (co-careldopa 25/100: carbidopa 25 mg/100 mg levodopa) tablets. Following this, he has a reasonably good period before the next dose is due. He is also taking Sinemet CR two tablets t.d.s. and ropinirole 3 mg t.d.s.
What is the nature of his new symptom?

82 i. This patient with frontal balding, facial diplegia and proximal and distal limb weakness, most probably has MMD. MMD is a neurogenetic disorder characterized by muscle weakness and wasting associated with myotonia and other systemic abnormalities. It is inherited in an autosomal dominant manner.

ii. The best way to confirm your diagnostic impression is to do a neurologic examination and DNA testing. Check for grip and percussion myotonia. An EMG would also show myotonic discharges in addition to the presence of myopathic features. A DNA based test is available and highly specific. The disease is caused by an expansion of a CTG repeat in the *MMD* gene on chromosome 19.

iii. There are many systemic complications of this disease. Cardiac involvement (often a conduction defect) with cardiac arrhythmias is seen in more than half the patients. Cataracts in the anterior and posterior subcapsular zones are frequent. Diabetes and glucose intolerance are probably secondary to insulin resistance. Other endocrine problems can include hypogonadism and thyroid dysfunction. Smooth muscle involvement may cause gastrointestinal dysmotility and gallbladder disease.

83 Dyskinesia. When commencing levodopa therapy for parkinsonism, patients are generally started on 1 Sinemet-Plus or 1 Madopar 125 t.d.s. These drugs consist of a combination of levodopa and a peripheral DOPA decarboxylase inhibitor to prevent inappropriate peripheral activation to dopamine. Over the years, the doses of these drugs are usually gradually increased in amount and frequency as the underlying disease worsens. Dyskinesias are a common late side effect of such levodopa therapy. About 10% of patients per year of therapy will develop dyskinesias, involving uncontrollable choreoathetoid movements and dystonic posturing. Controlled release preparations may be given once at night to help with nocturnal or early morning 'off' symptoms, or may be given 2–3 times a day alone or in combination with straight levodopa in an effort to smoothen fluctuating symptoms.

Some physicians may instead commence therapy with controlled release preparations of levodopa to minimize dose fluctuations that are thought to have a particular tendency to result later on in dyskinesia, but there is no clear evidence for this protective effect. Dopamine agonists, such as pergolide, ropinirole and cabergoline may be used on their own or in addition to levodopa for similar reasons, or simply for added anti-parkinsonian action. However, they are usually less powerful than levodopa when given in doses that avoid side effects such as nausea or psychosis.

84 With regard to the patient in 83, do you alter his medical management (e.g. reduce or increase the immediate release levodopa or controlled release levodopa; change the pergolide; increase or decrease the frequency of his immediate release or controlled release levodopa; or none of the above)?

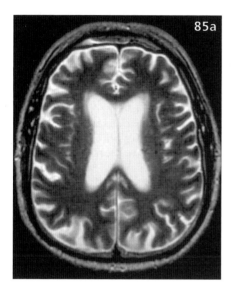

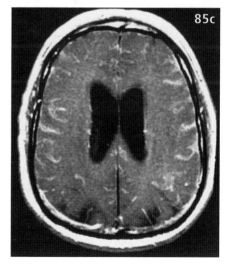

85 A 74-year-old chronic alcohol user was found obtunded with a WBC 19,900/µl and 90% neutrophils. These MR images were obtained (**85a–c**).
i. Which MR sequences are shown?
ii. What is the likely diagnosis? How do the imaging findings support it?

84 There is unfortunately no simple therapeutic solution to combating dyskinesias. However, a number of general guidelines should be noted. (1) The severity of dsykinesia is dose-dependent and so a balance has to be struck between 'off' symptoms of bradykinesia and rigidity and 'on' dyskinetic symptoms (patients usually prefer to be slightly dyskinetic than to be 'off'). (2) Regular controlled release levodopa more than twice a day tends to accumulate and to cause troublesome dyskinesias. (3) Dyskinesias may also occur in relation to dramatic fluctuations in levodopa levels rather than to high peak levels; the solution in this situation is to place the patient on a higher dose of longer acting medication instead of reducing the total levodopa level. However, accumulation may then occur. Sometimes the best compromise is in fact achieved with large but infrequent doses of normal release levodopa. The patient will rapidly come 'on', minimizing coming-on dyskinesia and will then at least enjoy some periods of good quality 'on' during the day.

Amantadine, a drug with relatively mild anti-parkinsonian action, seems to be rather effective in reducing dyskinesias in combination with existing therapy. Difficult cases may eventually be considered for a continuous infusion of subcutaneous apomorphine or intragastric levodopa. Deep brain stimulation or lesioning in the globus pallidus or in the subthalamic nucleus is becoming another established alternative. Pallidal procedures may reduce dyskinesias, while subthalamic procedures may have a greater anti-parkinsonian action, and allow a reduction of the dyskinesia-inducing medication. Note that deep brain lesioning or stimulation is unlikely to improve the non-dyskinetic features of anti-parkinsonism beyond the patient's current best-quality 'on' state.

In the case described above, the patient probably has coming-on dyskinesia. The best management may therefore be to increase rather than decrease the Sinemet-Plus doses, to reduce the controlled release levodopa frequency, and perhaps to add amantadine.

85 i. Three sequences are shown: T2-weighted (**85a**), FLAIR (**85b**), and T1-weighted with gadolinium (**85c**).
ii. The imaging diagnosis is meningitis. The T2-weighed image shows mild cerebral volume loss and enlarged ventricles but is otherwise unrevealing (**85a**). FLAIR images are similar to T2-weighed images, in that they show parenchymal edema and other pathologic processes as areas of increased signal intensity, but differ from T2 sequences in that signal from normal intraventricular and sulcal CSF is suppressed. CSF in the sulci is normally dark on FLAIR sequences. When CSF protein is increased due to meningitis or hemorrhage, it becomes bright, resembling the appearance of CSF on T2-weighted images. In this case (**85b**), the FLAIR images indicated proteinaceous CSF within the sulci and was supported by the results of a subsequent lumbar puncture. CSF protein was markedly elevated at 35.6 g/L (3.56 g/dl). T1-weighted images after administration of gadolinium (**85c**) show marked lepto-meningeal enhancement and mild hydrocephalus, one complication of purulent meningitis. CSF and blood cultures ultimately yielded *Staphylococcus aureus*.

86 A 27-year-old male with insulin-dependent diabetes mellitus presents with neck pain and some numbness into his fingertips bilaterally. WBC count is elevated to 17,000 and an ESR is 64. The radiograph (86) shows destruction of vertebral bodies from C3–5. What is the likely diagnosis?
(a) Metastatic carcinoma.
(b) Vertebral osteomyelitis due to *Pseudomonas* species.
(c) Discitis due to *Staphylococcus aureus*.
(d) Fracture dislocation of C3/4.
(e) Vertebral osteomyelitis.

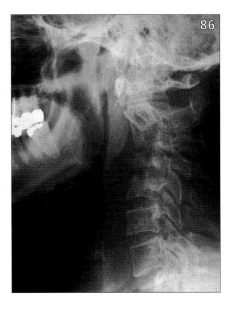

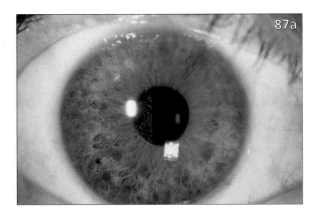

87 A 37-year-old female presents with complex partial seizures. Examination of her eyes reveals abnormalities of the iris (87a).
i. What are the abnormalities shown, and what other abnormalities would you look for?
ii. How is the condition inherited?
iii. What could be the cause of her epilepsy?

86 (e). The radiograph clearly show destruction of vertebral bodies which extends across the endplates and disc spaces and results in their collapse. This is likely to be from infection and that belief is supported by the laboratory data. The most common organism that causes vertebral osteomyelitis or pyogenic spondylitis is *Staphylococcus aureus*. Intravenous drug users have a higher incidence of infection with *Pseudomonas* than other populations which are predisposed to osteomyelitis, but *S. aureus* is still the leading organism.

87 i. These are Lisch nodules, hamartomas within the iris. They are a pathognomonic feature of NF1. Other cutaneous features of this condition are cutaneous neurofibromas (**87b**), plexiform neurofibromas, café-au-lait spots, and axillary freckling. Hypertension can result from renal artery stenosis or pheochromocytoma.

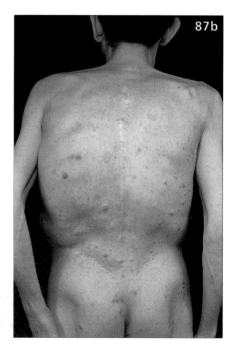

ii. NF1 is inherited as an autosomal dominant condition with abnormalities in the *neurofibromin* gene on chromosome 17.

iii. The incidence of CNS tumors especially optic nerve glioma is increased in NF1. In addition, there is an increase in the incidence of cortical dysplasia in NF1.

88 A 26-year-old Indian female presented with a 3-month history of malaise, headache and a slowly progressive right-sided hemiparesis. A coronal gadolinium-enhanced MRI is shown (88).
i. What abnormalities are seen?
ii. What is the most likely diagnosis?
iii. What other features may be present with this diagnosis?
iv. How should this patient be treated?
v. List other possible causes of the MRI appearances.

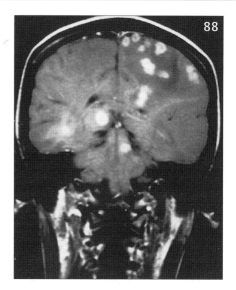

89 A 70-year-old male falls from his golf cart and strikes his forehead on the cart path. There is no loss of consciousness though he does sustain a laceration to the forehead. Following the event he complains of some minor neck pain with radiation into the occiput. However, he says that his hands feel fine and there is no evidence of motor weakness on examination. After closing the laceration, his neck pain is still present and it increases with any movement of his neck. A lateral radiograph is shown (89).
What is the diagnosis?
(a) Type III odontoid fracture.
(b) Jefferson's fracture.
(c) Type II odontoid fracture.
(d) Os odontoideum.
(e) Type I odontoid fracture.

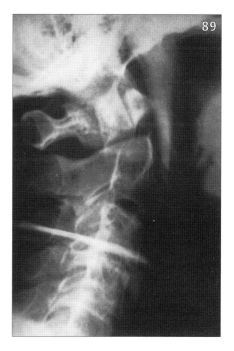

88 i. Multiple ring enhancing lesions in the cerebral cortices bilaterally (predominantly on the left) and one lesion in the left side of the pons. There is edema associated with the superficial left-sided cerebral lesions with effacement of the sulci and lateral ventricle on the left.

ii. The most likely diagnosis is TB (multiple tuberculomas are evident).

iii. Other features that may be present are: meningism, hydrocephalus, seizures, pyrexia, weight loss, night sweats, lymphadenopathy/cold abscess, previous or current pulmonary TB, SIADH, Addison's disease picture secondary to adrenal involvement.

iv. (1) Quadruple anti-tuberculous therapy with pyridoxine cover for 3 months and triple therapy continued for 1 year to 18 months. Classically, this would include isoniazid, rifampicin, pyrazinamide and either ethambutol or streptomycin; however, with more prevalent resistance other antibiotics are being increasingly used. The pyridoxine prevents the development of an isoniazid-induced peripheral neuropathy. Ethambutol can cause optic neuropathy and blindness, and regular ophthalmologic reviews are essential while on the drug. (2) Corticosteroids for 3–6 months. There is some controversy over the use of steroids. The symptoms can be exacerbated initially with steroid use.

v. Other possible causes are: cerebral metastases (although edema is usually associated with each lesion); bacterial abscesses, e.g. septicemia/endocarditis; cerebral toxoplasmosis; neurocysticercosis (the scolex of the tapeworm is usually visible in the center and inactive cysts become calcified, which would be black on MRI); cryptoccocoma – this presentation would be unusual. Usually, the picture is of meningitis with microabscess formation.

89 (c). The plain film reveals a displaced fracture across the base of the dens. This is referred to as a type II odontoid fracture and is the most common fracture of the C2 vertebral body. Type III fractures are the next most common and extend into the base of the C2 vertebral body. Type I fractures are very rare (not seen or <5% in all series) and involves a fracture of the very tip of the odontoid process, well above the base. Os odontoideum is a chronic condition resulting in hypermobility at the C2 vertebral body, presumably due to a non-healed odontoid fracture. A Jefferson's fracture is a three or four part fracture of the C1 ring.

90 As work-up and treatment are proceeding for the patient in 89, he acknowledges that he has had no previous trauma to his neck, that his health has been good except for some minor hypertension which is well controlled, but he does smoke half to one pack of cigarettes per day.

What is the best treatment option for this man?
(a) Soft cervical collar as needed.
(b) Surgical fusion with an odontoid screw.
(c) Hard cervical collar for 6 weeks.
(d) Halo bracing for 10–12 weeks.
(e) Halo bracing for 4 weeks.

91 A 53-year-old Indian male presented with progressive and painless loss of vision in the left eye over 3 weeks. The visual symptoms in the left eye seemed to be worse in the lower half of the field on standing up. One week later he began to notice weakness around both sides of his mouth and difficulty blinking. On examination, corrected acuities were 6/6 on the right and 6/36 on the left. The left monocular field was constricted with reduced color vision on that side. It was difficult to obtain clear views of the left fundus, the right fundus was normal. There was a left relative afferent papillary defect. There was bilateral facial weakness affecting all muscle groups. The MRI scan (91) is a weighted coronal scan after administration of gadolinium.

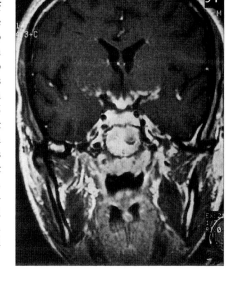

i. What does the MRI scan demonstrate?
ii. What is the clinical diagnosis?
iii. Why is the patient's vision worse after standing?
iv. What other investigations may help to confirm this?

90 (b). Although there has never been a randomized controlled trial of bracing versus surgery for the treatment of type II odontoid fractures, several studies point to several characteristics which yield a higher non-union rate. These include smoking, age >40 years, >5 mm (0.2 in) of displacement, or angulation >10°. This gentleman meets at least two of these criteria and the fracture is almost displaced 5 mm (0.2 in). Therefore if his surgical risk is low, operative fixation with either odontoid screw or posterior C1–2 fusion will yield the lowest pseudoarthrosis rate.

91 i. The MRI scan shows pathologic enhancement of the basal meninges.
ii. The patient has evidence of a left optic neuropathy as evidenced by reduced color vision and an afferent papillary defect. He also has bilateral lower motor neuron seventh nerve palsies. The combination of optic neuropathy, bilateral lower motor neuron facial weakness, involvement of the anterior vitreous and basal meningeal enhancement is highly suggestive of neurosarcoidosis.
iii. The difficulty in visualizing the left fundus suggests involvement of the anterior vitreous. If a large amount of cells are present in the anterior chamber they may form a precipitate which settles on standing, thus explaining the patient's position-dependent symptoms.
iv. The neuroophthalmologic appearances in sarcoid can often be diagnostic and patients should undergo a full neuroophthalmologic work up including a search for anterior and posterior segment disease, with slit-lamp examination and fluoroscein angiography, as well as seeking visual evoked potential evidence for optic nerve disease. Where possible tissue confirmation should be obtained to confirm the diagnosis. Kveim tests are no longer a recommended investigation, partly due to the scarcity of material but also the attendant risks of using splenic homogenate from patients with sarcoidosis.

CSF abnormalities are common in patients with neurosarcoidosis, with an elevation of CSF protein, a pleocytosis, and oligoclonal bands which are frequently matched in the serum. The sensitivity of CSF ACE levels are poor since this is frequently elevated when the protein content or cell count is elevated in the CSF. Whole-body gallium scanning remains a useful indicator of systemic disease. A plain chest radiograph, serum calcium and serum ACE should also be performed.

Treatment includes oral and i.v. pulsed steroids. Many patients require more aggressive immunotherapy with agents such as MTX and chloroquine (which requires ophthalmologic monitoring).

92 A 56-year-old female presented with a 2-month history of daily headaches. The pain was bifrontal, exacerbated by movement, sometimes throbbing and at other times described as a pressure sensation. The headache was provoked when erect, and accompanied by nausea and tinnitus. Significant relief was obtained on lying down. There had been no antecedent to the onset of the symptoms. She was not taking any medication. There was no previous history of headache and the past medical history was uneventful. Neurologic and general examination was normal.

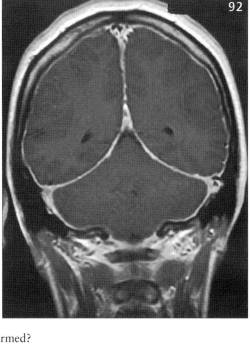

i. What investigation has been performed and what does it show (**92**)?
ii. What diagnosis should be suspected ?
iii. How could the diagnosis be confirmed?
iv. Give four possible therapeutic options.

93 This 62-year-old male has suffered a grade II SAH from this lesion demonstrated on cerebral angiography (**93**).
i. What is the diagnosis?
ii. What treatment would you choose and why?

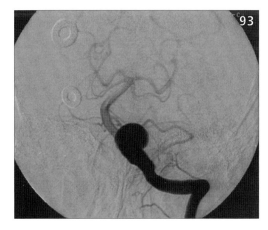

92 i. An MRI head scan with gadolinium enhancement shows diffuse meningeal enhancement.
ii. The history suggests intracranial hypotension. There is no preceding history of operative procedure, lumbar puncture, head or back injury or systemic ill-health, therefore a diagnosis of SIH should be considered. The hallmark of SIH is prominent headache with upright posture, improved with recumbency. The headache may be accompanied by nausea, vomiting, auditory and vestibular disturbances such as tinnitus and dizziness, and visual disturbance including sixth nerve palsy and visual field defects. A history of minor trauma or vigorous exercise has been reported in up to 50% of cases. Many patients improve spontaneously in 2–4 weeks. The symptoms may, however, continue for several months and in some patients, years. Recurrence is rare.
iii. Diffuse meningeal enhancement on MRI with gadolinium is the most consistent finding on imaging in patients with low pressure headache; there is no definitive evidence of inflammation on meningeal biopsy. Other described MRI findings include subdural hygroma and hematoma, tonsillar herniation, flattening of the pons and bowing of the optic chiasm over the pituitary gland. These abnormalities usually resolve with symptomatic improvement. The diagnosis can be confirmed by measurement of CSF pressure. This is usually ≤70 mm CSF pressure (≤9.3 kPa) with normal composition, although a mildly raised Hg and RBC count, and lymphocytic pleocytosis may be found.
iv. Current treatment of low pressure CSF headache includes bed rest, oral/i.v. fluids, and oral/i.v. caffeine. If conservative treatment fails, an epidural blood patch may provide symptomatic relief. Symptomatic relief has also been reported following infusion of intrathecal saline.

93 i. This is a vertebro-basilar dissecting aneurysm secondary to dissection of the blood into the subadventitial plane. Unlike subintimal dissections which present with ischemic symptoms, these present with bleeding and are more common in the posterior fossa.
ii. Direct surgery for this is no longer the treatment of choice. If the contralateral vertebral is robust, endovascular parent vessel occlusion is the simplest and safest option. If the contralateral vertebral is hypoplastic and test occlusion fails, stenting is an alternative though less attractive option given the chance of rupturing the vessel. Anticoagulation is not indicated.

94 The following physical findings are consistent with brain death *except*:
(a) Lack of oculocephalic or Doll's eye movements.
(b) Lack of oculovestibular or cold-water caloric testing.
(c) Triple flexion.
(d) Decerebrate posturing.

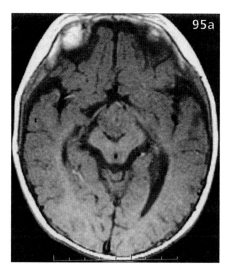

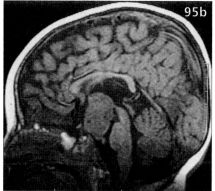

95 An 11-year-old male presents with precocious puberty and uncontrollable laughing episodes with subsequent generalization. Work-up includes a brain MRI (**95a, b**).
i. What type of seizures are these?
ii. What does the MRI show?
iii. Discuss the treatment options for this lesion.

96 In the recovery room a patient who has just undergone removal of a pituitary tumor develops confusion, a fever, and postural hypotension.
i. What is the possible diagnosis?
ii. What electrolyte abnormalities may be found?
iii. How can this disorder by treated?

94 (d) Decerebrate posturing. The clinical diagnosis of brain death refers to irreversible loss of all brainstem function, lack of consciousness, and no motor response to noxious stimuli. Examinations documented by two different examiners and the failure of spontaneous breathing off the ventilator (concomitant rise of pCO_2 = 60 mmHg [≤8 kPa] with the apnea test) are required for the determination of brain death. Use of neuromuscular blocking agents has to be excluded as prolonged muscle weakness may mimic lack of motor response with brain death. Cardinal features in the clinical determination of brain death include: fixed, unreactive pupils, lack of aversive eye movements on Doll's head maneuver (absent oculocephalic reflex), or tonic deviation of the eyes directed to the cold caloric stimulus (absent oculovestibular reflex); absent gag, cough, or evidence of corneal reflexes; motor unresponsiveness to deep noxious stimuli; and no spontaneous breathing above the ventilator set rate. Reflexes mediated solely by the spinal cord, deep tendon reflexes or triple flexion are compatible with brain death. The presence of brainstem mediated decorticate or decerebrate posturing is *not* compatible with brain death. Other exclusion criteria for brain death include severe hypothermia (below 32°C [90°F]) or electrolyte or acid-base abnormalities, intoxicating or sedative drugs, or endocrine crisis.

95 i. Laughing episodes with secondary generalization are known as gelastic seizures (partial complex seizures). Patients with gelastic seizures commonly have intellectual impairment and psychiatric disturbances.
ii. A hypothalamic (tuber cinereum) hamartoma. They are typically hypodense on T1-weighted MRI, hyperdense on T2-weighted MRI, and do not enhance. They lie between the infundibular stalk anteriorly and the mamillary bodies posteriorly. Histologically, they are benign lesions that resemble gray matter.
iii. Surgical options are considered only if the seizures cannot be adequately controlled with anti-epileptic medications. If possible, surgical resection is preferred. If not, gamma knife radiosurgery can also be used to treat these lesions.

96 i. These clinical findings are consistent with adrenal insufficiency or Addisonian crisis.
ii. Electrolyte abnormalities include hyponatremia, hyperkalemia and hypoglycemia.
iii. Treatment includes both a mineralocorticoid such as hydrocortisone and a mineralocorticoid such as desoxycorticosterone acetate or fludrocortisone. Methylprednisolone is not recommended for acute treatment.

97 This 39-year-old female has previously undergone mastoid and middle ear surgery for a vascular mass. She now presents with this follow-up angiogram (**97**).
i. What is the possible diagnosis?
ii. What anatomic landmarks should be identified to expose this lesion?
iii. What are the boundaries of Kawase's triangle and why is it important?

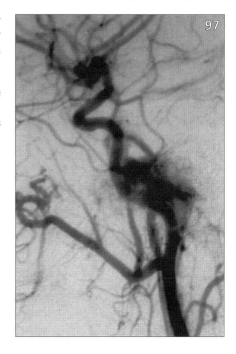

98 A 25-year-old male presented with a very slowly progressive 10-year history of clumsy feet, a tendency to fall and inability to run. Further questioning revealed that he had never been good at sports at school and had always run with a clumsy gait. One of his two sisters had a similar history as did his father. Nerve conduction studies showed a symmetrical, diffuse demyelinating neuropathy with the motor NCV of the right median nerve being 30 m/s. A picture of one of his feet is shown (**98**).
i. What is shown in this picture?
ii. What is the most likely diagnosis in this man?

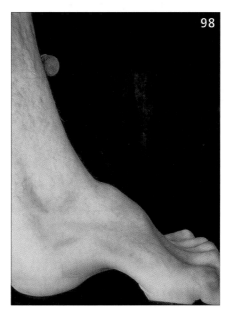

103

97 i. The angiogram shows a glomus tumor involving the horizontal portion of the petrous carotid artery.

ii. The horizontal portion of the petrous carotid artery can be exposed by extradural dissection beneath the GSPN and just medial to the middle meningeal artery, the eustachian tube and tensor tympani muscle. It lies with Glassock's triangle defined by the foramen spinosum, cochlea and V3 as it enters the foramen rotundum. The GSPN shows the carotid canal, tracing the middle meningeal artery back to the foramen spinosum or working anteromedially from the arcuate eminence reveals the GSPN. Care is needed in dissecting the GSPN because it is connected to the facial nerve at the geniculate ganglion. Proximally the petrous carotid can be followed through the petrous genu to the vertical segment. Distally it can be followed to its trigeminal segment beneath V3 and into the cavernous sinus. Additional exposure may be obtained by splitting the gasserian ganglion and trigeminal roots parallel to the nerve fibers between V2 and V3.

iii. Kawase's triangle is a pyramidal block of bone whose summit is the petrous apex. From the summit the edges are formed medially by the superior petrosal sinus at the petrous ridge, laterally by the greater superficial petrosal nerve that overlies the petrous carotid artery, and inferiorly by the inferior petrosal sinus in the occipito-petrous fissure. An imaginary line perpendicular to the middle fossa floor that contains the ICA forms the base. There are no important structures such as nerves or vessels in this region; therefore removal of this part of the petrous bone allows access to the posterior fossa from the middle fossa.

98 i. This picture shows pes cavus, a foot deformity seen relatively commonly when a chronic neurological condition such as a neuropathy is present during the first two decades of life.

ii. The most likely diagnosis in this patient is CMT 1A (HMSN 1A). This is the commonest form of CMT (HMSN). It is an autosomal dominant demyelinating neuropathy which usually presents in the first two decades of life with mild motor problems in the feet. The commonest signs are hyporeflexia, mild distal weakness and sensory loss and foot deformity. Nerve conduction studies confirm a demyelinating neuropathy with the median nerve motor NCV being <38 m/s. Sural nerve biopsy shows a hypertrophic demyelinating neuropathy with Schwann cell onion bulb formation. The commonest underlying genetic abnormality in this disease (accounts for 90% of cases with CMT 1) is a 1.5 Mb duplication of chromosome 17p11.2 which contains the gene *PMP-22*. Point mutations of *PMP-22* can more rarely cause this form of CMT 1, called CMT 1A or HMSN 1A. Another rarer form of autosomal dominant CMT 1 is CMT 1B (HMSN 1B) due to point mutations in the human *Po* gene on chromosome 1. There is an X-linked form of CMT 1 (CMT X1) in which carrier females are much less severely affected than affected males. This is due to mutations in connexin 32, a gap junction protein on the X chromosome. The other common form of CMT is CMT 2 (HMSN 2) which is an axonal neuropathy and usually autosomal dominant. No genes have been determined for this type of CMT but linkage to chromosomes 1, 3 and 7 have been described. *Po* mutations can rarely present with the CMT 2 phenotype.

99 A 64-year-old male complained that he was having increasing difficulty naming objects and with language function in both English and his native Arabic. Apart from an obvious nominal dysphasia and a mild comprehension deficit his speech was fluent with normal articulation, prosody and syntax. There were no abnormalities of memory function. Bedside cognitive testing showed impaired verbal fluency, but normal praxis skills, cognitive estimates and bimanual alternating movements of the hands.

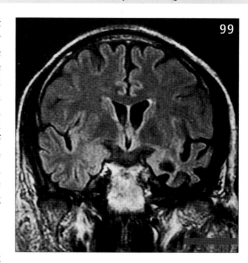

i. What does the MRI scan show (99)?
ii. What is the differential diagnosis?
iii. What is the most likely underlying pathology?

100 A 16-year-old male is referred to you with complaints of headache, nausea, and intermittent vomiting which have increased over the last 2 months. After handing you his recent contrast MRI (100), his parents emphasize the memory difficulties he has had over the past several months. His physical examination is remarkable for ataxia and Parinaud's syndrome.

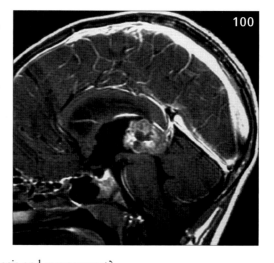

i. What is Parinaud's syndrome?
ii. What does the MRI show?
iii. Give a differential diagnosis for this lesion.
iv. What additional tests might you want to assist with both diagnosis and management?

99 i. The MRI scan shows marked atrophy of the left temporal lobe.
ii. The differential diagnosis includes one of the frontotemporal syndromes – fronto-temporal dementia, primary progressive aphasia, or semantic dementia – or Alzheimer's disease. Since episodic memory was intact, Alzheimer's disease is unlikely to be present. There were no symptoms or signs of a frontal lobe disorder such as personality change to indicate a frontal lobe dementia. Radiologically, in Alzheimer's disease the mesial temporal atrophy tends to be symmetrical bilaterally, whereas in semantic dementia, as in this case, the atrophy is asymmetrical with greater left-sided involvement with an anterior–posterior gradient.
iii. Tau positive and argyrophilic Pick bodies. Alternatively, focal degeneration characterized by neuronal loss, gliosis, and mild spongiform changes (or 'non-specific focal atrophy').

100 i. Parinaud's syndrome is a convergence, accommodation, and an upward gaze palsy often with lid retraction. Patients may also have fixed pupils (dissociated light–near response) and nystagmus retractorius. It is common in patients with masses causing direct pressure on the quadrigeminal plate (e.g. pineal tumors) and in patients with hydrocephalus

Markers associated with tumor types			
	AFP	β-HCG	PLAP
Germinoma	–	–	+
Teratoma	+	–	–
Endodermal sinus (yolk sac)	+	–	+/–
Embryonal carcinoma	–	–	+
Choriocarcinoma	–	+	+/–

AFP: alpha fetoprotein; β-HCG: beta human chorionic gonadotropin; PLAP: placental alkaline phosphatase

causing compression of the mesencephalic tectum by a dilated suprapineal recess.
ii. The MRI demonstrates a heterogeneously enhancing mass in the pineal region causing lateral and third ventricular enlargement.
iii. Statistically, the most likely tumor in this patient is a germinoma. However, many different tumors can be seen in the pineal region. They include other germ cell tumors (e.g. choriocarcinoma, endodermal sinus tumor or yolk sac tumor, embryonal carcinoma, and teratoma), pineal gland tumors (e.g. pineocytoma, pineoblastoma), glial tumors (e.g. astrocytoma, glioblastoma, ependymoma, and oligodendroglioma), or other miscellaneous tumors including meningioma and metastasis.
iv. Germ cell tumors characteristically (but not always) give rise to tumor markers beta-HCG and AFP in the CSF. Elevated CSF beta-HCG is classically associated with choriocarcinomas, but also occurs in a minority of germinomas. AFP is usually elevated in endodermal sinus tumors and embryonal carcinomas. When positive, these markers can be followed and used to assess treatment and recurrence. Because many pineal region tumors have mixed cell types, these markers alone are usually not sufficient for definitive diagnosis (*see table above*).

101 With regard to the patient in **100**:
i. What type of hydrocephalus (communicating or non-communicating) does he have?
ii. Discuss the treatment options for this patient's hydrocephalus.

102 An HIV positive male with a CD4 count of 50 cells/mm^3 presented with a 4-day history of back pain, followed by the development of weakness of his legs. By the time of admission he was incontinent of urine. On examination he had a flaccid paralysis of the legs with grade 3 power proximally and grade 0 distally. The knee and ankle reflexes were absent and the plantars unreactive. Pin prick sensation was reduced to the mid thigh on the right and the mid shin on the left. A MRI scan of the thoraco-lumbar spine was normal. CSF examination showed: WBC 60/mm^3 (90% neutrophils); protein 1.1 g/L (0.11 g/dl); sugar 3.2 mmol/L (57.7 mg/dl); blood sugar 6.3 mmol/L (113.5 mg/dl).
i. What is the differential diagnosis?
ii. What is the most likely cause?
iii. What other tests or examination will help confirm the cause?

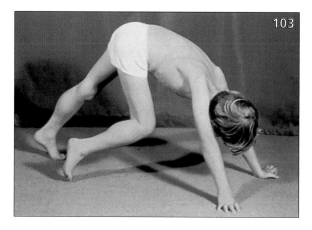

103 This 9-year-old male with calf hypertrophy and a creatine kinase of 5,000 units was diagnosed as having DMD (**103**).
i. What is the inheritance pattern of this disease?
ii. What is the life expectancy?
iii. What are the best methods for confirmation of the diagnosis?
iv. Why would you like to do DNA testing in this patient?

101 i. This patient has non-communicating (obstructive) hydrocephalus, because the CSF circulation is blocked where the tumor mass is compressing the cerebral aqueduct. This causes an increase in the size of the lateral and third ventricles, but the fourth ventricle remains normal because it is distal to the blockage. This is in contrast to communicating (non-obstructive) hydrocephalus, where CSF circulation is blocked at the arachnoid granulations, causing all the ventricles to be enlarged.
ii. There are three methods to treat this patient's hydrocephalus: (1) ventriculostomy; (2) ventriculo-peritoneal shunt; and (3) third ventriculostomy. Because this patient's hydrocephalus is chronic, the best choice is a third ventriculostomy. This treats the hydrocephalus immediately but allows time for further diagnostic work-up (e.g. tumor markers) before tumor resection. Furthermore, third ventriculostomy avoids the permanent nature of a shunt (a significant number of patients will not need a shunt after tumor removal) and prevents possible tumor seeding in the peritoneum. If the patient had presented with acute hydrocephalus, however, a ventriculostomy should be placed, followed by a definitive tumor resection within a few days.

102 i. The differential diagnosis of this lumbar polyradiculopathy syndrome in an HIV infected patient is lymphomatous infiltration, syphilitic meningoradiculitis, herpes simplex type 2 and CMV polyradiculopathy.
ii. The finding of a neutrophil pleocytosis suggests that CMV is the likely cause. In such cases the MRI scan may be normal or may show thickened nerve roots.
iii. PCR for CMV DNA. CSF cytologic examination will help exclude a lymphomatous process but repeated CSF examination may be required. There may be evidence of CMV infection elsewhere and therefore a careful examination of the retina is necessary.

103 i. DMD is a disorder inherited in an X-linked recessive manner. The location is chromosome Xp21. Deletions in the gene result in a deficiency or absence of a protein called dystrophin.
ii. DMD is characterized by progressive proximal weakness with pseudohypertrophy of the calves. There is also often myocardial involvement. The onset is usually before age 3 years and patients are wheelchair bound by age 12 years. BMD is allelic to DMD, having a defect in the same gene. BMD has a milder course. Dystrophin is reduced rather than absent in BMD. The life expectancy depends on whether the disorder is classical DMD or BMD. DMD has a shortened life expectancy with death in the 20s, usually secondary to respiratory failure or cardiomyopathy. A few patients may survive longer. Patients with BMD usually survive to a more advanced age.
iii. The best methods for confirming the diagnosis are: (1) a muscle biopsy, which shows signs of a myopathy and absent dystrophin staining of muscle fibers; (2) DNA testing which detects about 65% of mutations in the DMD gene.
iv. The DNA testing allows confirmation of the clinical diagnosis. It also provides a method for carrier detection in female relatives and may be used in prenatal diagnosis.

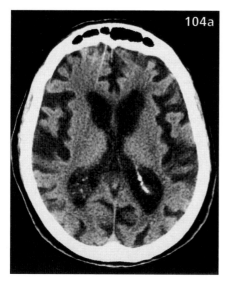
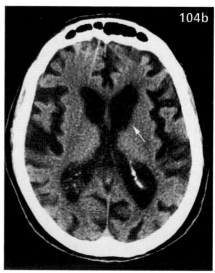

104 A 55-year-old female presented with longstanding dementia. Her mother and sister both died in their 40s with the same condition.
i. What are the CT findings (104a, b)?
ii. What is the differential diagnosis? Are there imaging findings that narrow the diagnostic possibilities?

105 A 45-year-old female with a past history of breast cancer treated with chemotherapy, lumpectomy and axillary radiotherapy presented to the ENT clinic with a 4-month history of increasing deafness bilaterally, ataxia and facial weakness. She had lost 6.3 kg (14 lb) in weight.
i. What does the MRI scan (105) show?
ii. What further investigation should she now have?
iii. What are the treatment options?

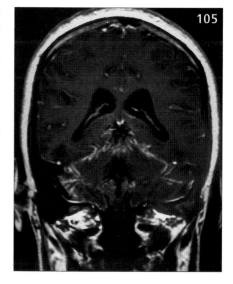

104 i. Nonenhanced CT (**104a**) shows marked prominence of both sulci and ventricles. The ventricular enlargement is proportional to the size of the sulci, indicating volume loss rather than hydrocephalus. For a patient of age 55 years, the brain is markedly atrophic. While overall volume loss is indeed present, the caudate heads normally indent the frontal horns of the lateral ventricles. In this case, the frontal horns are bulbous and laterally convex, indicating atrophy of the caudate in addition to generalized volume loss (**104b**, arrow).

ii. The differential diagnosis of age-inappropriate, generalized volume loss is broad and includes: dehydration, chronic ethanol abuse, steroid use, AD, post-traumatic volume loss, and multi-infarct dementia. Several conditions show more focal volume loss, or focal volume loss with generalized atrophy. These include: Huntington's chorea (caudate and putamen), Parkinson's disease (substantia nigra), progressive supranuclear palsy (midbrain), and chronic ethanol or dilantin toxicity (cerebellum). The focal caudate atrophy in this case, along with the family history of early dementia and death suggests Huntington's chorea. This patient had characteristic choreiform motions on physical examination.

105 i. Diffuse leptomeningeal enhancement around the cerebellum and brainstem and communicating hydrocephalus consistent with malignant meningitis.

ii. CSF examination with cytology looking for the presence of malignant cells.

iii. Cranioradiotherapy, with or without intrathecal MTX. This can be administered either via an Omaya intraventricular reservoir or via repeated lumbar punctures. The hydrocephalus may be treated with a ventriculo-peritoneal shunt. Corticosteroids are useful for controlling the inflammatory response.

Malignant meningitis whereby the leptomeninges (pia mater and arachnoid) are infiltrated by tumor is increasingly common, particularly in breast cancer, leukemia/lymphoma and melanoma. Sometimes the CNS is the sole site of relapsed disease. The clinical presentation is variable but most commonly consists of symptoms and signs of raised ICP, cranial nerve palsies, gait ataxia and neck/back pain. Diagnosis is usually by repeated lumbar punctures, which show malignant cells in up to 90% of cases. Even if abnormal cells are not seen the CSF is almost always abnormal with an elevated opening pressure, WBC count and protein concentration. CSF glucose is reduced in up to 30% of cases. Brain and spine MRI scans show meningeal enhancement and hydrocephalus in about 60% of patients. The prognosis is very poor with average survival of 1–2 months although occasional long term survivors are reported, particularly with breast cancer.

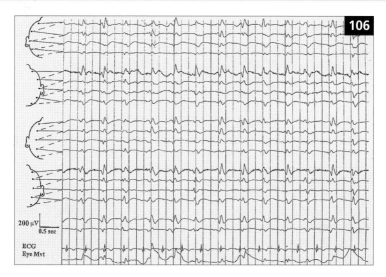

106 A 57-year-old lady was referred for an urgent EEG (106). She had been admitted to a psychiatric hospital 3 weeks earlier with recent-onset depression.
i. What are the main EEG abnormalities?
ii. What is the diagnosis?

107 Below which level would a drop in CBF lead to electrocerebral silence on EEG and coma?
(a) 55 ml/100 g brain tissue/min.
(b) 25 ml/100 g brain tissue/min.
(c) 15 ml/100 g brain tissue/min.
(d) 8 ml/100 g brain tissue/min.

108 A 48-year-old healthy male was involved in a roller-blading accident and sustained abrasions of his left knee, shin, and foot, which did not require suturing. Four days after the accident, he began to experience severe progressive aching and burning pain that was not alleviated by ibuprofen or acetaminophen. Approximately 2 months later, in addition to his pain, he began to notice swelling of his left foot, accompanied by glossy smooth, and cold skin.
i. What is the diagnosis in this patient?
ii. What is the most effective treatment strategy?

111

106 i. The record consists of generalized continuous periodic sharpened diphasic and triphasic waveforms, recurring at intervals of 0.3–0.6 seconds. The intervening background consists of no recognizable rhythms, with loss of the normal waking background activity. This patient had a very rapid onset of dementia and myoclonus.
ii. This record is virtually diagnostic of CJD. Myoclonic jerks may occur in association with the periodic sharp-waves.

107 (c) 15 ml/100 g/min. CBF normally ranges from 50–60 ml/100 g brain tissue/min. CBF levels <25 ml/100 g/min result in EEG changes and impaired consciousness. Below 15 ml/100 g/min CBF, there is disappearance of the spontaneous brain electrical activity on EEG and coma. CBF <10 ml/100 g/min results in irreversible cell damage with massive efflux of potassium and neuronal cell death.

108 i. The described pain syndrome is that of classic RSD, or using a more recent classification scheme, CRPS type I. CRPS-I is a sympathetically-maintained pain that may be caused by blunt trauma (which may be trivial), medications, inflammatory disorders, burns or frostbite, and immobility following cerebral or myocardial infarction. While the mechanisms involved in CRPS-I have not been fully elucidated, both peripheral (sympathetically-induced sensitization of sensory receptors, abnormal afferent sympathetic discharges) and central (sensitization of spinal nociceptive neurons) nervous systems have been implicated.
ii. Treatment strategies are outlined (*see table below*). It is important to note that patients should be treated as early as possible because early treatment is the most important predictor of future pain relief. For a healthy 48-year-old one may try a lumbar regional anesthetic block, and if successful, proceed with surgical interruption of the lumbar sympathetic ganglia. In a more medically unstable patient a more conservative route is preferred, consisting of physical therapy, TENS, trigger point injections, and intravenous regional blockade.

Treatment strategies

Treatment modality	Comments
Anesthetic interruption of regional sympathetic ganglia	Stellate, celiac, lumbar
Surgical sympathectomy	For patients who have reproducible but temporary positive effects from anesthetic blockade
Intravenous regional blockade under tourniquet isolation	Sympathetic blocking agents such as phentolamine, reserpine, guanethidine
Oral sympatholytic medications	Propranolol, phenoxybenzamine, prazocin
Other medications	Anti-inflammatory agents, narcotics, anti-convulsants, calcium-channel blockers, tricyclic antidepressants
Electrical stimulation	Epidural dorsal column stimulation, TENS

109 A 39-year-old Caucasian female attorney/barrister with complaints of fatigue and weight gain is referred to your clinic for evaluation. Her past medical history is unremarkable. How-ever, she describes to you that she easily gets upset (more so than usual) and that she stopped men-struating 4 months ago. She is concerned about 'early meno-pause', and has noticed that she tans more easily recently. Physical

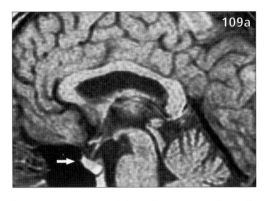

examination reveals a hypertensive, heavy-set woman, with ecchymoses and purple stria on her lower lateral abdomen bilaterally. An imaging study of the patient is shown (109a).
i. What specific laboratory test do you need to confirm your suspected diagnosis?
ii. What is the most appropriate treatment?

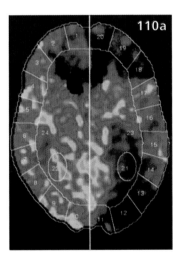
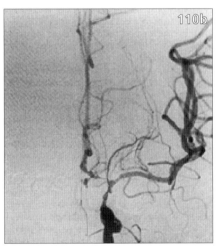

110 A 61-year-old female presents with grade I SAH. She underwent successful clipping of an Acom aneurysm and was intact post-operatively. Then on day 4 she developed increasing lethargy. Her CT scan was normal but her xenon CT (110a) and her angiogram (110b) were not.
i. What is the diagnosis?
ii. What is the medical treatment?
iii. If despite this the patient continues to deteriorate what procedure might you consider and when?

109 i. Cushing's disease describes the clinical entity of Cushing's syndrome secondary to an ACTH secreting pituitary adenoma. In addition to the signs and symptoms listed (**109b**), patients with Cushing's disease can also have hyperpigmentation of the skin and mucous membranes due to the melanin stimulating hormone cross reactivity of ACTH. The MRI shown (**109a**) demonstrates a normal appearing pituitary gland (arrow), consistent with the observation that up to 50% of pituitary tumors are ≤5mm (≤0.2 in) at the time of diagnosis. In addition to a baseline endocrine work-up there are specific laboratory tests used to confirm the diagnosis of Cushing's disease as the source of endogenous cortisol (**109b**).
ii. The most appropriate treatment for this patient is trans-sphenoidal surgery, with an expected cure rate of 80%. For medically unstable patients unable to tolerate surgery, alternative treatments include radiation and/or medical therapy.

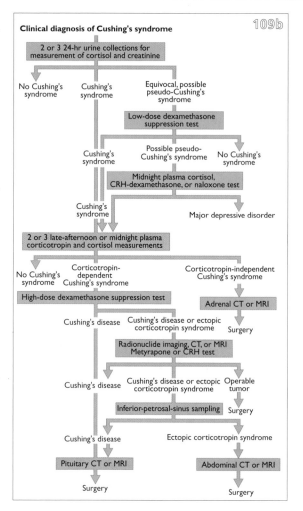

110 i. Cerebral vasospasm.
ii. Hypertensive, hypervolemic therapy with hemodilution to a hematocrit of 30. Nimodipine is also given.
iii. Balloon angioplasty should be considered for spasm of the proximal A1, M1, vertebral, basilar and ICA. For distal spasm intra-arterial papavarine is an option. Either should be instituted as soon as it is determined that the patient is medically refractory.

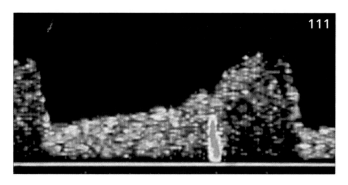

111 This TCD abnormality is seen during a CEA (111).
i. What does it represent?
ii. How can it be prevented?
iii. What is the correct sequence to apply and remove arterial clamps during CEA?
iv. What techniques and what findings can be used to detect hemodynamic insufficiency during CEA?

112 This patient has a renal transplant, is on cyclosporin and is immuno-compromised. The acute illness of confusion and fever has evolved over 1 week. The MRI is shown (112).
i. What is the likely diagnosis?
ii. What is the treatment?
iii. What is the prognosis?

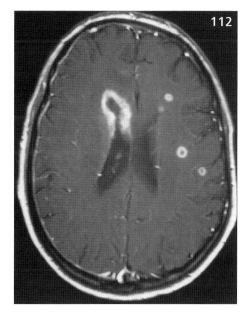

111 i. This TCD finding represents a DMES and is associated with cerebral emboli.
ii. Emboli may be prevented by: (1) aspirin continued in the peri-operative period; (2) avoiding dissection along the posterior wall of the carotid; (3) administration of heparin (701 U/kg) 3 minutes before cross clamping (protamine is not given); (4) avoiding manipulation of the common carotid artery unless the ICA is clamped; (5) using an intraluminal shunt only if indicated and, when inserted, using meticulous technique; (6) continuously flushing the carotid artery with heparinized irrigation (4000 IU/L of normal saline) until the arteriotomy is repaired; (7) before final closure of the arteriotomy allowing back-bleeding through the ICA. Re-occlude the ICA and then permanently remove the superior thyroid occlusion for constant back-bleeding as the closure is finalized.
iii. The correct sequence of arterial clamp application is: internal, common, and then external carotid. The correct sequence of arterial clamp removal following carotid endarterectomy is: external, common, and then internal carotid. This sequence prevents any embolic material from going into the internal carotid circulation; instead it is flushed through the external carotid artery.
iv. The critical threshold for irreversible intra-operative ischemia is a CBF of 18–20 ml/100 g/min. Intra-operative rCBF measurements, however, are rarely used. Instead, techniques such as EEG monitoring, compressed spectral analysis, SSEP monitoring, TCD, or measurements of stump pressure are used to detect hemo-dynamic insufficiency during CEA. EEG monitoring or compressed spectral analysis reliably correlate with CBF; moderate changes may be observed when CBF is between 10–18 ml/100 g/min, and major changes when CBF is <10 ml/100 g/min.

Major changes consist of attenuation of 8–15 Hz activity to minimal or nil and at least a twofold increase in delta activity. Moderate changes include persistent 8–15 Hz whose amplitude is reduced by at least 50% and an increase in delta activity. When CBF is >25 ml/100 g/min EEG changes are usually not seen. SSEP monitoring provides similar physiologic information to EEG but is less frequently used.

TCD may predict safe occlusion time in minutes using the formula: (100VcMCA/VoMCA) where VcMCA = middle cerebral artery velocity when the ICA is closed and VoMCA = middle cerebral artery velocity when the ICA is open. A MCA mean velocity <30 cm/s or <30% of pre-occlusion velocity suggests that carotid occlusion may not be safely tolerated, whereas a VMCA <10 cm/s is associated with a CBF of 10 ml/100 g/min. Finally, a stump pressure >50 mmHg (6.7 kPa) is considered safe. However, isolated measurements are not reliable, and stump pressure measurement has been largely replaced by evaluation of physiologic function.

112 i. The features are classical of cerebral aspergillosis with cerebral and ependymal lesions seen on MRI.
ii. Systemic and intrathecal antifungal chemotherapy.
iii. The prognosis is extremely poor. Eradication is usually impossible and obstructive hydrocephalus complicates management in many cases.

113 A 63-year-old otherwise fit male presented with bilateral, sequential, severe subacute visual loss.
i. What does the MRI (113) show?
ii. What is the most likely diagnosis?
iii. What are the further management and prognosis?

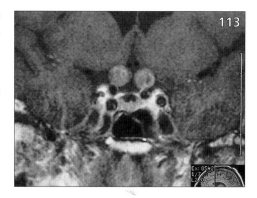

114 A 37-year-old HIV positive male presents with a 1-week history of headache and progressive left-sided weakness. On examination he is alert and orientated. He has a left homonymous hemianopia and pyramidal weakness affecting the left face, arm and leg with hyperreflexia and bilateral extensor plantar responses.
i. What is the differential diagnosis of the abnormality on the T_2 MRI brain-scan (114)?
ii. What blood tests and what other investigations may help in making a diagnosis?
iii. How should he be managed?

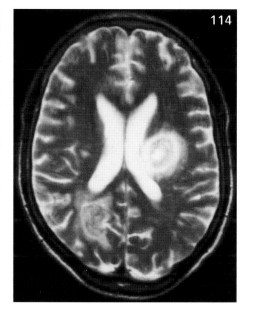

115 A 65-year-old right-handed female developed sudden onset of disabling and persistent tremor of her right hand and arm. She has since been unable to work or perform chores as a result. There is no family history or drug history. On examination, she has an irregular coarse slow jerky tremor of the right upper limb. It is present at rest and on posture and action. When performing mental arithmetic the tremor subsides in severity. No other neurologic deficit is identified.
   Give a differential diagnosis.

113 i. The MRI shows markedly enlarged optic nerves, the so-called 'shotgun barrel' appearance.
ii. The most likely diagnosis is malignant glioma. Sarcoid may also produce such intrinsic disease of the anterior visual pathways, but usually with marked gadolinium enhancement also involving the cerebral meninges.
iii. Malignant glioma of the anterior visual pathway is diagnosed by biopsy, which usually shows a malignant (grade IV) astrocytoma.
iv. Radiotherapy is often given but has no definite effect on outcome. The majority of patients die within 1 year of diagnosis.

114 i. The differential diagnosis in an HIV positive patient with a low CD4 count lies between toxoplasmosis, primary CNS lymphoma, and tuberculoma.
ii. If the toxoplasma serology is positive, this means the patient has been exposed to the organism and is vulnerable to reactivation when immunosuppressed. Over 95% of toxoplasmosis in HIV is a reactivation rather than *de novo* infection. A MRI may be helpful since a single lesion on MR is more likely to be lymphoma. More recently, thallium-201 SPECT scans have been utilized – lymphoma showing increased uptake relative to toxoplasma abscesses.
iii. The standard treatment is to treat patients with anti-toxoplasma drugs such as sulphadiazine and pyrimethamine plus folinic acid for at least 2 weeks. If there is a significant response the diagnosis is one of toxoplasmosis. If the patient deteriorates a stereotactic brain biopsy should be considered. The patient continued to deteriorate. A brain biopsy showed primary CNS lymphoma.

115 This woman has psychogenic tremor. Features in the history suggestive of phychogenic tremor are a previous history of psychiatric or physical disease, a sudden onset and a functionally or socially limiting manifestation. Clues on examination include variable characteristics, distractibility, inability to maintain the tremor while simultaneously tapping voluntarily with another limb, and association with other inexplicable or inconsistent neurologic abnormalities. The differential diagnosis in this case would primarily include a vascular or vasculitic episode, rubral tremor and dsytonic tremor. A vascular event, perhaps involving the thalamus or other diencephalic structures, may result in sudden onset unilateral coarse tremor. So-called rubral tremor, arising from the brainstem and sometimes related to small cell bronchial carcinoma, is characteristically associated with presence at rest and upon posture and action. Dystonic tremor may be unilateral, variable, coarse, and show distractibility, and is occasionally not associated with any other features of dystonia.

A wider differential of tremors that may sometimes be confused with psychogenic tremor also includes essential tremor, parkinsonian tremor, cerebeller ataxic tremor, primary orthostatic tremor, paraproteinemic neuropathy, drug effects (e.g. lithium), hyperthyroidism, rhythmic neuroleptic side effects (e.g. mouth and tongue tremor), and rhythmic manifestations of myclonus or symptomatic dystonic mixed movement disorders, such as those found in Wilson's disease or in systemic lupus erythematosis.

116 With regard to the patient in 115, what investigations may be appropriate?

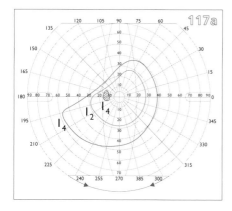

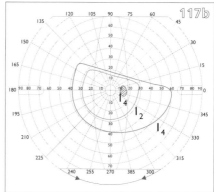

117 Visual field testing of a 56-year-old male showed predominantly supero-temporal field loss bilaterally (117a left eye, 117b right eye).
i. Where is the likely site of the disease process?
ii. What should be done next?

118 A 17-year-old male presents with a short history of complex partial seizures with postictal dysphasia. Examination is unremarkable.
i. What does his MRI show (118)?
ii. What would be your management plan?

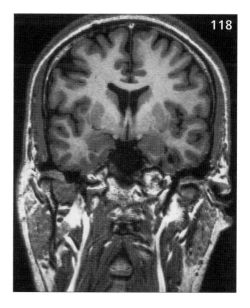

116 In this case, an MRI scan of the brain would be indicated to look for a vascular event or other symptomatic cause of tremor. Blood investigations for vasculitic and connective tissue disease would be appropriate. Neurophysiologic studies provide further information. As well as identifying peripheral lesions, they distinguish different tremor forms. A pyschogenic tremor oscillation will have a single generator that will be interfered with by simultaneous voluntary generation of rhythmic movements while organic tremor will be unaffected by such voluntary activity. In addition, essential and dystonic tremors run independently in different body parts. Although primary orthostatic tremors is linked between body parts in the same way as psychogenic tremor, the bursts are too rapid to be 'voluntarily' reproduced. The bursts of rhythmic myoclonus are similarly often too brief for generation through voluntary pathways.

117 i. The visual field defects comprise a pseudo-bitemporal hemianopia, sloping across and not respecting the vertical meridian. The disease process is likely to be intraocular. The common causes for pseudo-bitemporal hemianopia are congenitally tilted optic discs, bilateral inferior retinal detachments, sectoral retinitis pigmentosa, and excessive eyelid skin (dermatochalasis).
ii. An ophthalmologic assessment should be arranged. There is no need to perform imaging of the optic chiasm.

118 i. The MRI shows an intrinsic cortically-based lesion of mixed signal intensity. There is no discernible effect on adjacent brain tissue. In view of the normal examination, seizure location in the temporal lobe of mixed constitution, and the lack of effect on adjacent structures, it is most likely to be a DNT. The differential diagnosis includes another developmental lesion or a low-grade glioma.
ii. He requires counseling and treatment for his epilepsy. Lifestyle issues must be addressed specifically, e.g. he may recently have acquired a provisional driving licence. Anti-epileptic drug treatment will be required; monotherapy should be the aim. With respect to the underlying lesion, he requires careful monitoring. DNTs are hamartomatous lesions, with a very low likelihood of change or intralesional hemorrhage. The associated epilepsy is often, but not always, refractory to drug treatment, but the associated epilepsy is likely to be controlled by surgical resection. However, in this case, presurgical assessment will need to take into account seizure semiology given the location of the lesion. Chemotherapy or radiotherapy are not indicated in the management of DNTs. The differential diagnosis includes a low-grade glioma. In the absence of evidence of local pressure effects, monitoring of the lesion clinically and with serial MRI (initially at 6 monthly intervals while the patient displays no neurologic signs or symptoms other than stereotyped epileptic seizures) would suffice. If the patient's seizures remain medically refractory, epilepsy surgery is warranted.

119 A 48-year-old female gave a 2-year history of severe bioccipital throbbing headaches radiating frontally, precipitated by coughing, sneezing, bending or lifting. The onset was sudden with rapid resolution after 15–30 minutes. There were no additional features to the headache for which she had taken simple analgesics, pizotifen and amitriptyline without good effect. Clinical examination was normal.

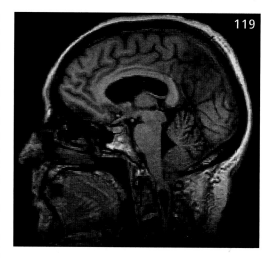

i. With what type of headache does the patient present?
ii. What does the MRI scan (119) show? Are the headache and MRI abnormality related?
iii. Had the neuroimaging been normal what diagnosis would you give the patient? What treatment may provide symptomatic relief in this situation?

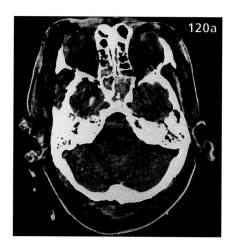
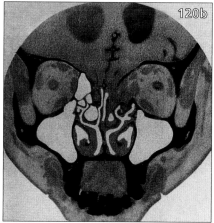

120 The head CT scans shown here (120a, b) were performed after a female noted clear fluid intermittently draining from her nose. She had been in a motor vehicle accident several weeks earlier.
i. What do the head CTs show?
ii. Describe the typical diagnostic work-up for this entity.
iii. What is the usual treatment?

119 i. The patient gives a typical description of cough headache. Cough headache is characterized by severe head pain precipitated within seconds by coughing, sneezing, lifting, straining or any other valsalva maneuver. The headache is usually bilateral and of short duration, typically from seconds up to 30 minutes.

ii. The MRI scan shows a type I Arnold–Chiari malformation accompanied by a syrinx. Symptomatic cough headache is usually caused by lesions of the posterior fossa and include basilar impression (e.g. Paget's disease of the skull), space occupying lesion (e.g. meningioma), midbrain cysts and Arnold–Chiari malformation. Individuals with Arnold–Chiari type I malformations may present with headache as the only symptom. However clinical examination should look for evidence of raised ICP, cerebellar syndrome, syringomyelia or a combination of disorders of the cranial nerves, medulla, cerebellum and spinal cord. Although cough headache may initially be an isolated feature of the disorder, most patients ultimately develop further symptoms and abnormal neurologic signs (usually within 5 years).

iii. A diagnosis of benign cough headache is made on the characteristic clinical history described, in the absence of intracranial disease. The syndrome is more commonly seen in men in the age range 40–80 years. The symptoms ultimately improve or resolve spontaneously in the majority of individuals. Relief may be obtained with indomethacin and some patients have responded to therapeutic lumbar puncture. Patients with symptomatic cough headache tend not to respond to indomethacin.

120 i. The head CT (**120a**) demonstrates intracranial low density consistent with air. This is indicative of a skull base fracture where CSF is able to exit and air enter the intracranial compartment via the sinuses.

ii. In cases where CSF is leaking without significant pneumocephalus, the first line of treatment is often lumbar drainage. Diversion of CSF allows the leak to seal. If it persists, it is important to identify the exact site of leak so it can be repaired. Persistent leak is often associated with meningitis and headache. Coronal head CT through the skull base will often show the defect. Intrathecal contrast may improve the diagnostic efficacy in difficult cases (**120b**). Nuclear medicine studies can also be useful when no clear anatomical defect is identified.

iii. Treatment of a skull base defect associated with a CSF leak usually involves a craniotomy with dural repair and/or repair of the skull base defect with bone and fascia lata. Post-operative CSF diversion is routinely employed. Sometimes, defects can be repaired in a less invasive manner using trans-sinus or endoscopic techniques.

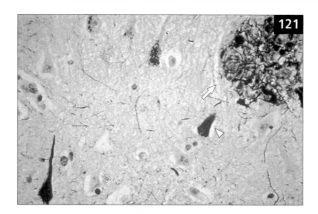

121 A 52-year-old female died with a 6-year history of progressive dementia. The figure shows microscopic changes of her cerebral cortex (121, arrow = tangle, arrowhead = plaque).
i. What is the diagnosis?
ii. There is a positive family history of early onset (before age 60 years) dementia in her father and paternal uncle. What are the likely causes of this syndrome?

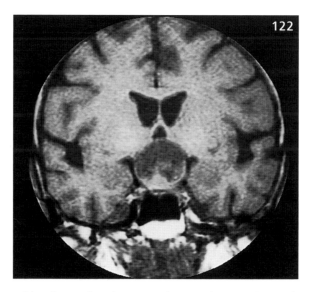

122 A 50-year-old male is referred to your clinic with a complaint of impotence and decrease in his peripheral vision. An imaging study of the patient is shown (122). Laboratory tests reveal a prolactin level of 1,500 µg/L (1,500 ng/ml).
What is the most likely diagnosis and the appropriate treatment?

123

121 i. The neuropathology shows intraneuronal neurofibrillary tangles and a neuritic amyloid plaque. She has AD. This is characterized by an adult-onset progressive dementia. Memory loss is associated with diffuse cerebral cortical atrophy. The neuropathology findings are microscopic A-beta amyloid neuritic plaques, intraneuronal neurofibrillary tangles and amyloid angiopathy. AD is the most common cause of dementia in North America and Europe. Most cases have late onset (after age 65 years) and are sporadic. About 25% of patients have a positive family history. A few cases have early onset before age 65 years. Familial cases have clinically and pathologically the same phenotype as sporadic cases.

ii. The patient has a positive family history of dementia with an age of onset before age 60 years. She has EOFAD. This rare disorder is transmitted in an autosomal dominant manner. There are four possible subtypes. The most common of the EOFAD, has a mutation in the *presenilin 1* gene at chromosome 14q24. A less common type has a mutation in the *APP* gene at chromosome 21q21.3-q22. A very rare type has a mutation in the *presenilin 2* gene at chromosome 1q31q42. Families with familial AD with no known mutations in these three genes have also been described. The only commercially available test for EOFAD screens for mutations in the *presenilin 1* gene.

122 Prolactin secreting adenomas can cause prolactin-induced menstrual disturbance and galactorrhea in women and symptoms of hypogonadism such as poor libido or impotence in men. The MRI (**122**) demonstrates a mass in the pituitary gland with compression of the optic chiasm (consistent with the patient's decrease in peripheral vision). The prolactin level of 1,500μg/L (1,500 ng/ml) should be interpreted as a significant elevation, attributable to a prolactin secreting adenoma (normal levels <25 μg/L [25 ng/ml] and stalk effect between 25–150 μg/L [25–150 ng/ml]). Prolactin secreting tumors are very responsive to dopamine agonists. The most appropriate treatment for this patient would be the prescription of a dopamine agonist such as bromocriptine followed by careful monitoring of the patient's response. Transsphenoidal surgery for decompression of the lesion should be considered only if the patient does not respond to or cannot tolerate medical therapy.

123 A 65-year-old female experienced sudden onset of severe headache and lost consciousness. She awoke several minutes later complaining of a headache and stiff neck. A CT scan of the head was normal.
i. What is the cause of loss of consciousness in this patient?
(a) Syncope due to severe pain.
(b) Severe migraine headache.
(c) Rapid rise in ICP.
(d) Asystole.
ii. Which of the following tests would be most useful for the diagnosis of SAH?
(a) An MRI scan.
(b) Repeat CT scan 12 hours later.
(c) Determination of RBCs in CSF.
(d) Spun CSF for xanthochromia.

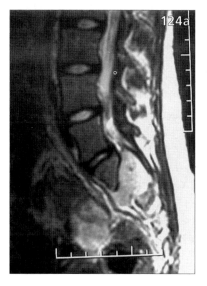

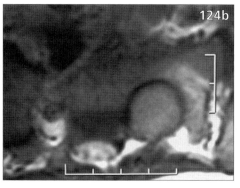

124 A 15-year-old female presents with a 9-month history of pain radiating down her left leg and numbness and tingling on the top of her foot. On examination, she has weakness of her left great toe. An MRI is ordered and is shown (**124a, b**).
i. Give a differential diagnosis for this lesion.
ii. Additional work-up includes an MRI of her thoracic spine showing two similar asymptomatic lesions. Give two syndromes this patient may have that would account for these lesions. What would you expect the pathology to be for each syndrome? What specific chromosomes would need to be analyzed for mutations?
iii. Outline a treatment plan for this patient.
iv. What is the risk of malignant degeneration for these tumors?

123 i. (c) Rapid rise in ICP.
ii. (d) Spun CSF for xanthochromia. The loss of consciousness seen in patients with SAH is believed to result from the forceful jet of blood emanating from a ruptured aneurysm that briefly but markedly increases ICP until it approximates MAP, leading to interrupted brain perfusion and syncope. The most sensitive test to confirm the diagnosis of SAH, when there is a strong clinical suspicion but negative initial CT scan, is examination of a freshly drawn, centrifuged specimen of CSF for xantho-chromia (straw-yellow color of the fluid). CSF xanthochromia develops between 12 hours and 2 weeks after the bleed, and can be found in up to 70% of patients after 3 weeks. The CSF typically clears of blood after centrifugation when there is traumatic tap.

124 i. The MRI (**124a, b**) demonstrates a homogeneously enhancing intradural, extramedullary mass. The differential diagnosis for this lesion would include nerve sheath tumors (neurofibroma and schwannoma) and meningioma.
ii. A careful search for multiple lesions should be made whenever an intraspinal tumor is suspected to be a meningioma or nerve sheath tumor, because there is a strong association of multiple lesions with both NF1 and NF2. If the patient has NF1, the tumor is more likely to be a schwannoma. Multiple spinal neuro-fibromas, on the other hand, are more likely to be associated with NF2. The genetic mutations responsible for NF1 and NF2 lie on chromosomes 17 and 22, respectively.
iii. The treatment of choice is lami-nectomy and total tumor resection, if this

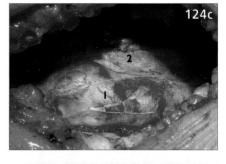

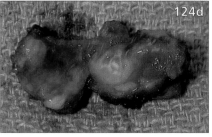

is possible (**124c**; 1 = tumor; 2 = normal dura). This patient had a schwannoma (**124d**). The symptomatic lesion should be resected immediately. The other tumors can be followed with serial imaging until they either show signs of progression or become symptomatic, at which time they should be resected.
iv. The risk of malignant degeneration is approximately 11% for these tumors.

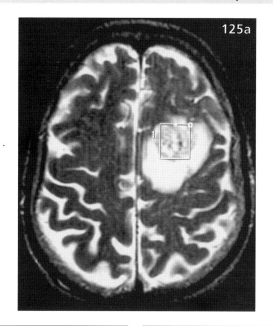

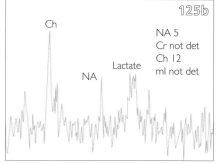

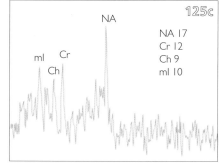

125 A 74-year-old right-handed surgeon presented with sudden onset aphasia.
i. What are the MRI and MR spectroscopy findings (125a–c)?
ii. Are they compatible with a diagnosis of primary brain neoplasm?

126 A 45-year-old male is referred to your clinic shortly after having bilateral carpal tunnel decompression surgery. He notes that his shoe size has increased significantly over the past year and that the gloves he bought just last winter do not fit his hands anymore.
What specific laboratory test do you need to confirm your suspected diagnosis?

125 i. An axial T2-weighted MRI (**125a**) shows a left frontal mass with surrounding high signal, vasogenic edema. MR spectroscopy obtained from the tumor (**125b**) and the contralateral normal white matter (**125c**) show that Ch and lactate are increased within the mass, and that NA is decreased. MR spectroscopy is a technique for analyzing the chemical composition of a specified brain region. It measures amounts of several metabolites including NA, myo-inositol, Ch, creatine, lactate, as well as lipids and other amino acids.

ii. In normal brain, NA, a marker for normal neurons, is elevated relative to Ch, a marker for cell membrane turnover. In patients with high grade tumors, Ch is increased and NA is decreased. In this case, considerable lactate is present as well, indicating some degree of necrosis. While these MR spectroscopy findings could indicate either a high grade neoplasm or cerebral infarct, the MR imaging findings suggest a tumor. The patient underwent craniotomy with intra-operative motor and speech mapping, with removal of a glioblastoma.

126 The patient described demonstrates some of the classic features of acromegaly (table right). Not infrequently, the diagnosis of acromegaly may be missed, resulting in palliative procedures such as carpal tunnel decompression. The importance of making the appropriate diagnosis is underscored by the increased mortality rate among untreated acromegalics, secondary to serious systemic illness such as hypertension, diabetes, and cardiomyopathy. The diagnosis of acromegaly may be confirmed by documenting elevated levels of GH and IGF-I within the appropriate clinical context. Diagnostic levels of GH as well as other pertinent tests are shown in the table below.

Features of acromegaly

- Enlargement of soft tissues, cartilage and bones in the face, hands and feet.
- Coarse skin.
- Soft, doughy hands.
- Enlarged viscera – heart, liver, thyroid.

GH stimulates growth and plays a part in control of protein, fat and carbohydrate metabolism. Excess GH in the adult causes acromegaly.

In childhood, prior to fusion of epiphyses, GH excess causes gigantism.

GH levels are usually increased to >10 mU/L. Increased serum levels of insulin growth factor-1 enhances the effect of growth hormone on target organs. Hyperglycemia normally suppresses GH secretion. GH samples are taken in conjunction with blood glucose tolerance test. The lack of GH suppression after glucose administration confirms the presence of a tumor.

Tests for acromegaly	
Test	*Diagnostic criteria*
IGF-I level (required for diagnosis)	Elevated above age and sex matched normal range
GH suppression testing (supportive evidence)	Failure of GH to fall to <1.0 µg/L (1.0 ng/ml) during an oral glucose tolerance test
Random GH level	Persistently elevated levels are suggestive, but cannot be used alone for diagnosis

127 With regard to the patient in **126**, what are some treatment options for this patient (i.e. medical and surgical)?

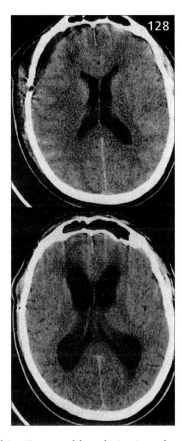

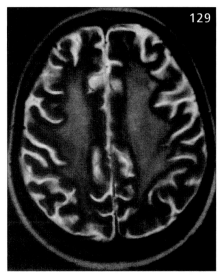

128 This 47-year-old male is 6 weeks post-clipping of an Acom aneurysm via a right pterional craniotomy (**128**). He was initially neurologically intact but has become increasingly confused over the past few days.
i. What is the diagnosis?
ii. What treatment would you choose?
iii. What other causes should be ruled out prior to treatment?

129 A 19-year-old female with acute lymphoblastic leukemia was treated with a combination of high dose systemic and intrathecal MTX, and prophylactic cranial irradiation. At second complete remission she was transplanted with a matched unrelated donor allograft. She was referred with behavior and personality change. She had become increasingly uncommunicative, incontinent of urine, and indifferent to her family. Her level of self-care had declined considerably. On examination she was almost mute, rigid, and had frontal release signs.
i. What does the MRI (**129**) show?
ii. What is the most likely cause?

Alternative medical therapies for acromegaly	
Medical therapy	**Efficacy**
Somatostatin analogs	
Octreotide (s.c. injection formulation)	Normalizes IGF-I levels in ~65% of patients
Depot formulations of octreotide (Sandostatin LAR Depot,)	Same efficacy as s.c. octreotide, but improved patient compliance
Dopamine agonists	
Bromocriptine	Normalizes IGF-I levels in ~20% of patients
Cabergoline	Normalizes IGF-I levels in ~30% of patients

Data from Freda PU and Wardlaw SL. Clinical Review: Diagnosis and treatment of pituitary tumors. *J Clin Endocrinol Metab* **84**:3859–3866, 1999.

127 Currently the best treatment for patients who can tolerate surgery is transsphenoidal decompression. Alternative medical therapies for those patients who are not surgical candidates as well as those who fail surgical treatment are outlined in the table above.

128 i. He has hydrocephalus, in part decompressed into the epidural space.
ii. This is best treated with a ventriculo-peritoneal shunt.
iii. Before treating, hyponatremia, vasospasm, drug toxicity and infection should be ruled out as possible contributing causes. A lumbar puncture can contribute to the diagnosis of communicating hydrocephalus.

129 i. Diffuse high signal change in subcortical white matter and cortical atrophy suggestive of leucoencephalopathy.
ii. The combination of previous MTX and cranial irradiation. The major delayed complication of MTX therapy is a leucoencephalopathy. It tends to occur in patients who have been treated for more than 6 months and is exacerbated by cranial radiotherapy, especially when administered before or during MTX therapy. Young women are particularly susceptible, even when given conventional doses. The clinical presentation is characterized by progressive cognitive impairment, behavioral changes and the development of akinetic mutism. CT/MRI scanning shows diffuse cerebral atrophy and white matter change. The clinical course is variable, with some patients stabilizing after discontinuation of the MTX while others rapidly progress to death (as did this patient). The cause is unknown and there is no effective treatment.

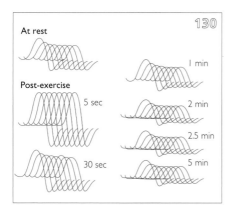

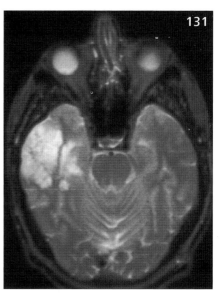

130 A 29-year-old lady was referred with difficulty swallowing for 2 months. She had noticed intermittent right-sided painless ptosis and double-vision over the previous year. Repetitive stimulation studies are shown (130). These are CMAP recordings from anconeus muscle following trains of 8 supramaximal stimuli at 3 per second to the nerve to anconeus. Trains recorded at rest, and at intervals following maximal voluntary contraction of the muscle for 20 seconds, are displayed.
i. What neurophysiologic phenomena are displayed?
ii. What is the diagnosis?
iii. What other neurophysiologic studies should be carried out?

131 A 27-year-old male presented with a 20-year history of temporal lobe seizures that had been resistant to medication. An MRI was performed (131).
i. What does the MRI show?
ii. What is the likely cause?
iii. What is the treatment?

132 A 55-year-old female presents with a 1-year history of quietness of voice and slowness of gait with frequent falls. She has a much longer history of urinary urgency that dates back to the delivery of her children. There is no family history or drug history. On examination, she has normal cognitive function, poor voluntary upgaze, a quiet monotonous voice, axial and distal rigidity and bradykinesia and upgoing plantar responses. Her gait is stooped with loss of arm swing. Postural reflexes are impaired.
  What is the diagnosis?

130 i. There is evidence of significant decrement at rest, with post-activation potentiation of <200%. There is also post-potentiation exhaustion, maximal 2–2.5 minutes after exercise.

ii. These findings are consistent with a postsynaptic neuromuscular transmission disorder, and in this clinical context are diagnostic of myasthenia gravis.

iii. Repetitive stimulation studies could also be carried out, recording from a facial muscle, e.g. nasalis. Single fiber EMG would detect increased jitter with fiber blocking. If a patient is on anticholinesterase inhibitor medication, this should be withheld the morning before assessment.

131 i. The MRI is a T2-weighted MRI (CSF is white, gray matter is lighter than white matter). This is usually better than T1 at showing pathology. In this scan there is a tumor in the temporal lobe with no associated mass effect.

ii. In view of the 20-year history of seizures beginning in childhood, and the MRI appearances, the tumor is almost certainly benign. In the past, these tumors were often categorized as 'low grade' gliomas, but recent histopathologic evidence has demonstrated that these tumors contain ganglioneuronal elements and are termed DNTs. These tumors commonly occur in the temporal lobes and result in temporal lobe epilepsy. They are often cystic on MRI or CT scan, and may be associated with cortical dysplasia.

iii. Surgical removal of a DNT has a high chance of resulting in remission of the epilepsy, even in cases where there is associated cortical dysplasia.

132 Multisystem atrophy. This is an acquired degenerative condition whose spectrum is quite broad and encompasses a number of named syndromes, namely striato-nigral degeneration (as in this patient), olivopontocerebellar atrophy and Shy–Drager syndrome. Individual patients may have elements of any or all of these subtypes. The features of the condition include a rather earlier mean age of onset than other akinetic-rigid syndromes, rapid deterioration, preserved cognitive function, cerebellar eye movement problems, bulbar dysfunction, stridor, axial and distal rigidity and bradykinesia, pyramidal dysfunction, cerebellar ataxia, anterior horn cell loss, early falls, urinary incontinence and autonomic dysfunction. The urinary dysfunction usually involves frank incontinence due to sphincter denervation. In women, trauma during vaginal delivery makes electrophysiologic demonstration of such denervation a much less specific finding. MRI may reveal cerebellar atrophy, low T2 intensity in the putamen and a cruciate pattern of abnormal signal in the brainstem. Pathologic examination, sometimes the only way to make a certain diagnosis, reveals oligodendroglial cytoplasmic inclusions.

133 With regard to the patient in **132**:
i. List the positive and negative features that make her more likely to have multi-system atrophy than other akinetic-rigid syndromes.
ii. What is the prognosis?

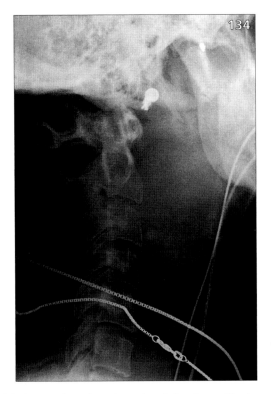

134 A 42-year-old skier is found at the side of the slope. She has no spontaneous respiration and fixed and dilated pupils. Following resuscitation, she is brought to the emergency department where a lateral radiograph of the cervical spine is performed as part of the trauma work-up (**134**). What is the likely diagnosis?
(a) Pulmonary embolus.
(b) MI.
(c) Occipital–cervical dislocation.
(d) Subdural hematoma.
(e) C3 fracture/dislocation.

133 i. The patient's early falls make idiopathic Parkinson's disease less likely. While supranuclear vertical gaze is a characteristic feature of Steele–Richardson syndrome, this is more specifically a downgaze problem, worse for voluntary than for reflexive eye movements. A mild upgaze problem is less specific and relatively common with increasing age. The condition is usually of older onset, and associated with cognitive impairment, axial more than distal rigidity, and a tendency to fall backwards rather than to be stooped forwards.

Corticobasal degeneration may be associated with dementia and typically begins with rigidity and loss of function in one arm, evolving into an 'alien' limb, where the arm makes random movements that the patient ignores. Other features include cortical sensory loss, apraxia, reflex myoclonus and athetosis.

Dementia with Lewy bodies could not be diagnosed in life without cognitive deficit or the condition's other features.

A mass lesion, such as a frontal meningioma, may result in a similar bradykinetic picture with mild pyramidal signs and must be borne in mind as an important differential diagnosis, but this presentation is relatively uncommon.

Even brief neuroleptic drug use can produce tardive dyskinesia later on which may appear as an akinetic-rigid syndrome, often with orofacial dyskinesias. A careful drug history should thus always be obtained.

Other rare causes of a progressive syndrome with akinetic-rigid features may include Huntington's disease, DRPLA, adult gangliosidoses, acaeruloplasminemia, Wilson's disease, neuroacanthocytosis, metochromatic leucodystrophy, NPD type C (type II S), neuronal intranuclear inclusion body disease, progressive pallidal atrophy (childhood-onset), lacunar infarctions, dementia pugilistica, postencephalitic parkinsonism, syphilis, prion disease, AIDS, AD and some frontotemporal dementias, Parkinson-dementia-ALS complex of Guam, and psychomotor retardation.

ii. The prognosis is poorer than in idiopathic Parkinson's disease, with patients expected to survive only 4–10 years from onset. There may be a response to levodopa, but this is usually temporary. There is a particular risk of death from respiratory arrest in some patients, which may be reduced if identified.

134 (c). The likely etiology of this person's demise given her age is trauma. While the radiograph does not show a fracture, it does reveal several centimeters of soft tissue swelling in the upper cervical spine (notice how far anterior the endotracheal tube is displaced) and a separation between the occipital condyles and the lateral masses of C1.

135 A 52-year-old female with MS (135) complains of symptoms consistent with TGN on both sides of her face. The arrows show periventricular white matter plaques.
i. How common is bilateral TGN?
ii. What are some of the etiologies of TGN?

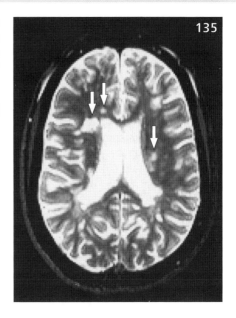

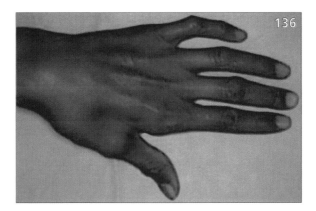

136 This 60-year-old male describes right-hand weakness (136). His cervical MRI is unremarkable.
i. What is the diagnosis?
ii. Where is the pathology and how can it be differentiated?
iii. What surgical options are available to treat this disorder?
iv. What is the surgical importance of the arcade of Struthers?

135 i. The annual incidence of TGN is 40 per million. The disease can occur bilaterally in up to 12% of patients. Eighteen percent of patients presenting with bilateral symptoms have MS. This incidence decreases to 2–8% in patients with unilateral symptoms.

ii. The identifiable etiologies of TGN include MS with demyelinating plaques within the brainstem, intracranial tumors, and vascular compression of the trigeminal nerve at the root entry zone. With respect to intracranial tumors, <1% of patients with facial pain harbor a tumor. Those with a tumor usually have atypical neuralgia, especially if the tumor is located outside the posterior fossa. These patients respond poorly to medical therapy. The vascular compression syndromes can be due to a vein, or more commonly, an artery. These are typically the SCA or, less commonly, the AICA, vertebral artery, or a persistent primitive trigeminal artery originating as a branch of the ICA.

136 i. There is wasting of the first dorsal interosseous muscle and hand intrinsics, consistent with a diagnosis of ulnar neuropathy.

ii. The most likely entrapment site is in the cubital tunnel at the elbow or in Guyon's canal at the wrist, which can be differentiated with careful EMG and NCV studies. In addition, patients with ulnar nerve entrapment at the wrist do not have sensory deficits on the dorsum of the hand because the sensory nerve to this region leaves the ulnar nerve in the forearm.

iii. There are several surgical approaches to disorders in the cubital tunnel: including medial epicondylectomy, simple decompression, subcutaneous transposition of the ulnar nerve, intramuscular transposition of the ulnar nerve, or submuscular transposition of the ulnar nerve. Simple decompression and transposition procedures are the most frequently performed operations. No randomized study has compared these two procedures; clinical series however, suggests that surgical results are comparable. These same series suggests that transposition is the preferred procedure when the symptoms have been prolonged (>1 year), there is recurrent subluxation of the ulnar nerve, valgus deformity of the elbow and muscle wasting is found.

iv. The arcade of Struthers is a fibrous septum located where the ulnar nerve passes through the medial intermuscular septum into the posterior compartment and is found about 8 cm (3 in) proximal to the medial epicondyle. Following anterior transposition of the ulnar nerve it may become a proximal tether; it is therefore important to release this fibrous tissue to prevent secondary compression.

137 A 28-year-old obese female presents to the emergency department with complaints of intermittent headaches and transient visual 'blackouts' lasting only a few seconds. On physical examination, she weighs 110 kg (244 lb) and is neurologically normal. A non-contrast head CT is normal except for slightly small ventricles (**137a**).

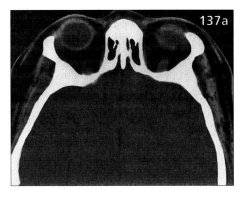

i. What is the most likely diagnosis, and what diagnoses must be ruled out?
ii. What are the next steps that must be taken to confirm your diagnosis, and what are the findings likely to be?
iii. What is the most important morbidity of this disease? List medical and operative strategies that may be used to treat this patient.

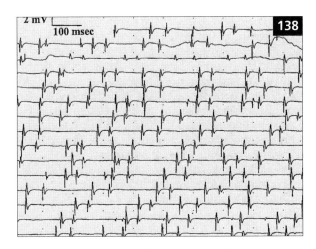

138 This 63-year-old lady was referred for assessment of progressive numbness of the lateral 4 digits of the left hand, with aching in the left upper arm. She had a carcinoma of the left breast treated 16 years previously. SNAP amplitudes from the left median nerve were significantly reduced without slowing across the wrist. This is a recording of CNEMG activity from the left APB muscle at rest, in raster display (**138**).
i. What abnormalities are evident?
ii. What diagnosis do they indicate in this case?
iii. What is the likely clinical outcome?

137, 138: Answers

137 i. The most likely diagnosis is IIH, or pseudotumor cerebri. This is a disorder characterized by symptoms and signs of increased ICP – including headache, transient visual disturbances, and papilloedema – but with no evidence of a mass or hydrocephalus. Pseudotumor cerebri is a diagnosis of exclusion, and the following processes must be ruled out: true mass lesions (e.g. tumor or hematomas), cranial venous outflow impairment (e.g. sinus thrombosis or congestive heart failure), infection, inflammatory conditions (e.g. neurosarcoidosis), vasculitis, metabolic abnormalities (e.g. lead poisoning), meningeal carcinomatosis, and complex migraines.

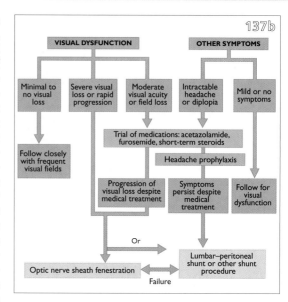

ii. After an imaging study is performed (CT or MRI), a lumbar puncture and a complete ophthalmologic examination should be performed. The opening pressure must be elevated above 20 cmH$_2$O, and CSF studies must be normal (protein may be slightly decreased) to fulfil the criteria for pseudotumor cerebri. Ophthalmologic examination reveals papilloedema in nearly all cases, an enlarged blind spot with concentric constriction of peripheral fields in the majority of cases, and visual field defects in some patients.

iii. Vision loss is the only major morbidity of this disease, so treatment is directed toward preventing this. A treatment algorithm for the management of IIH is shown (137b). No treatment has been subjected to prospective randomized studies. However, medical strategies that should be tried first include weight loss, fluid and salt restriction, diuretics (acetazolamide or furosemide), and short-term steroids. Surgical treatment is required in patients who develop progressive visual loss despite adequate medical therapy. The options include a lumbo-peritoneal shunt (or other shunt procedure) and optic nerve sheath fenestration. Other treatment options (not included in the algorithm) include serial lumbar punctures (often very difficult in obese patients) and weight reduction surgery.

138 i. There were persistent recurrent discharges at rest, often occurring as couplets and triplets.

ii. These findings are consistent with radiation brachial plexopathy. The discharges were myokymia-like, and their presence was strongly in favor of the brachial plexopathy being due to radiation rather than tumor infiltration. The differentiation between these conditions can be very difficult clinically.

iii. Plexopathy can develop months or years after radiotherapy, and it is usually progressive.

139 A 20-year-old male was referred to outpatient's with a 5-year history of pins and needles and weakness in his left hand, which had gradually spread up his arm, down into his leg and was now affecting his gait. In addition he was aware of constant neck pain which woke him at night. On examination he had profound weakness and wasting of his upper limbs with a mild asymmetric spastic paraparesis.

i. What does the MRI scan (**139**) show?
ii. What is the differential diagnosis?

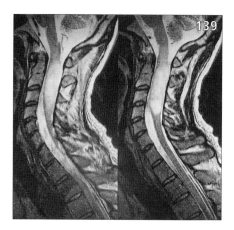

140 A 25-year-old HIV positive male with a past history of pulmonary tuberculosis, *Pneumocystis carinii* pneumonia and CMV retinitis was admitted with a 1-week history of fever and headache. He had been prescribed erythromycin prior to being admitted. The cranial CT scan was normal (**140a**). The CSF showed 110 cells/mm³ WBC (40% neutrophils and 60% lymphocytes); protein 1.75 g/L (0.175 g/dl); glucose 0.8 mmol/L (14.4 mg/dl); blood sugar 6.9 mmol/L (124.3 mg/dl).

i. What are the causes of meningitis in such a patient?
ii. What other tests should be performed on the CSF and blood?
iii. Three days after admission his condition deteriorated; he became increasingly drowsy and complaining of worsening headache. What are the possible causes?

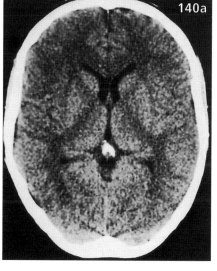

139 i. An enlarged swollen cervical cord mixed signal characteristics suggestive of an intramedullary spinal cord tumor.
ii. Cervical astrocytoma or ependymoma. Primary spinal cord tumors are rare neoplasms and occur more commonly in children. Most are benign. The most common early symptom is local pain along the spinal axis characteristically worse on lying down (thought to be due to venous congestion). Other symptoms include weakness paresthesias, radicular pain and occasionally sphincter disturbance. Children may present with delayed walking and scoliosis. MRI scanning with gadolinium enhancement is the imaging modality of choice. Surgery on cervical tumors is often limited to a biopsy and decompression because of the high risk of tetraplegia. Tumors in the conus, filum terminale and cauda equina can be excised en-bloc. Radiotherapy may be useful in about 50% of patients.

140 i. The causes of meningitis include those found in non-immunocompromised individuals – *Streptococcus pneumoniae, Haemophilus influenzae* and *Neisseria meningitidis.* Since the patient was treated with erythromycin prior to admission, a partially treated bacterial meningitis needs to be considered. However, in the immunosuppressed patient the other causes of meningitis include *Cryptococcus neoformans, Listeria monocytogenes, Histoplasmosis capsulatum,* and *Mycobacterium tuberculosis.*
ii. The specific tests for cryptococcal meningitis are staining with the Indian ink preparation which will reveal the fungi in 75% of cases, and measuring the cryptococcal antigen titers which will be positive in over 90%.

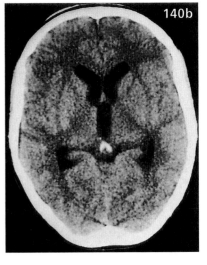

140b

Culture will be positive in 85%. The CSF should be stained with ZN even though this is a rather insensitive method for the diagnosis of tuberculous meningitis. The fluid should be cultured in the Löwenstein–Jensen medium with Kirchner enrichment or other medium such as BACTEC. The use of PCR techniques is still controversial and requires formal validation – the sensitivity varies from 48–100% with a specificity of 100%. In any HIV infected patient a CD4 count is a useful guide as to the etiological causes depending on the degree of immunosuppression.
iii. A deterioration may be due to: the development of an abscess, though one would expect some focal neurology; hydrocephalus due to a basal meningitis as in tuberculosis; or obstruction of the arachnoid villi in cryptococcal infection; seizures, the development of hyponatremia due to inappropriate ADH secretion; stroke due to an associated vasculitis. This patient had tuberculous meningitis diagnosed on ZN staining and subsequently developed an obstructive hydrocephalus (**140b**) that required shunting. The CD4 count was 70 cells/mm^3.

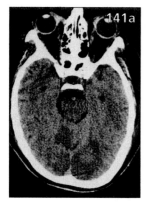
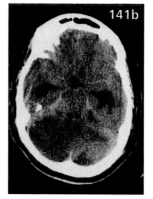
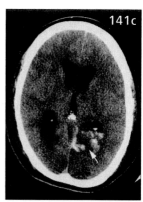

141 A 44-year-old female involved in a motor vehicle accident had this non-enhanced CT (141a). On the second hospital day, she remained comatose and a second CT (141b, c) and xenon CBF study (141d) were obtained.

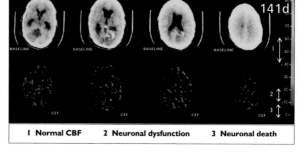

| I Normal CBF | 2 Neuronal dysfunction | 3 Neuronal death |

i. What does the initial CT show?
ii. What is the patient's prognosis based on the second CT examination and xenon CBF study?

142 A 17-year-old snow boarder takes a jump off a 7.7 m (25 ft) cliff at one of the local ski resorts, falls, and is unable to regain standing following several attempts. After transfer to the local emergency department he is noted to have two-fifths strength in hip flexion and quadriceps but no motor function in other lower extremity muscle groups. His upper extremity examination shows normal strength. On sensory examination, he has some sensation to light touch in his left leg as well as across the sacrum and perineum. His likely diagnosis is:
(a) T3/4 fracture dislocation.
(b) T12 burst fracture.
(c) L4 burst fracture.
(d) Type II sacral alar fracture.
(e) C7 burst fracture.

141 i. The admission nonenhanced CT
(141e) shows increased density in the basilar
artery (arrow), suggesting thrombotic
occlusion. In addition, decreased density in
the vascular territory of both posterior cerebral arteries and the right superior cerebellar
artery (arrowhead) indicates occlusion of the
basilar artery, or embolization from the
basilar or vertebral arteries. In the setting of
trauma, vertebral artery dissection is the
probable cause.
ii. Nonenhanced CT examinations (141b,
c) obtained 24 hours after the injury show
bilateral cerebellar infarcts, hemorrhagic
transformation of the left PCA territory
infarct (arrow), cerebral swelling, and acute
hydrocephalus. These findings confirm
evolution of infarcts in territories supplied

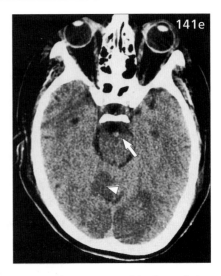

by the vertebrobasilar circulation, as well as complicating edema and hydrocephalus
due to compression at the level of the fourth ventricle or cerebral aqueduct.

The xenon CBF study is a recently developed CT technique for quantitatively
measuring CBF (141d). Four levels of the brain are repeatedly scanned while the
patient breathes xenon gas. The rate of increase in CT density of the brain reflects the
local CBF, which can be measured and displayed as a color map. Normal CBF is
50 ml/100 g/min. Brain tissue becomes ischemic and neuronal function is impaired at
flow <20 ml/100 g/min. Cellular death occurs when CBF is lower than
10 ml/100 g/min. In this case, CBF is 0–10 ml/100 g/min, indicating absent cerebral
perfusion and brain death. The xenon CT can be used to assess regional perfusion in
patients with cerebrovascular disease, vasospasm, and to adjust ventilation
parameters in trauma patients with impaired cerebral autoregulation.

142 (b). Given the mechanism of axial load after a fall from a height, the most likely
diagnosis is a fracture at the thoraco-lumbar junction with an injury to the conus
medullaris. This is the most common location of fracture in the thoraco-lumbar spine.
Fractures in the lower lumbar spine (L3–5) are much less common and can often
result in surprisingly little neurologic deficit due to the ability of the cauda equina to
accept more deformation than the spinal cord. Fracture/dislocations in the upper
thoracic spine (T1–T10) are often the result of very high mechanism injuries (thrown
from a high-speed vehicle) with a high degree of complete paralysis. Sacral alar fractures also result from motor vehicle accidents, and occur in conjunction with pelvic
fractures and result in asymmetric deficits.

143 A 38-year-old female presented with sudden-onset dysarthria, and weakness of the left arm and leg. The symptoms lasted several hours before gradual resolution. When seen the following day general and neurologic examination was normal. She gave a history since her teens of attacks of migraine without aura and on occasions with typical visual aura. Her current presentation had not been accompanied by headache. The patient had a history of stroke in several family members. However, she had recently undergone a medical examination for insurance purposes and no cerebrovascular risk factors had been identified.

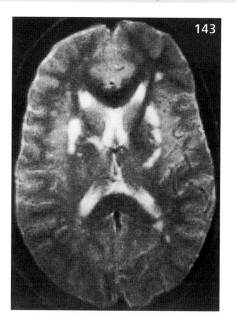

i. What does the patient's MRI head scan (143) show?
ii. What diagnosis should be considered from the history and results of the imaging?
iii. What is the prognosis?

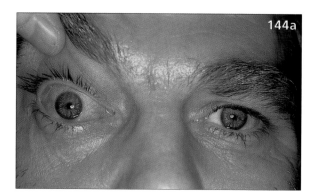

144 A 50-year-old male was knocked out by a fall down a flight of stairs. Upon waking he was found to have a complete right ptosis, and generalized limitation of movements of the right eye.
i. What other clinical features are shown (144a) and what is the diagnosis?
ii. What other clinical features would confirm this diagnosis?
iii. How might the vision of the right eye be affected?
iv. What is the further management?

143 i. The MRI shows leucoencephalopathy – prominent white-matter hyperintense signal changes on T2-weighted images.
ii. CADASIL.
iii. The main clinical presentation of CADASIL is of recurrent subcortical ischemic strokes with progressive subcortical dementia, migraine with typical aura, and major mood disturbances characterized by depression which may alternate with manic episodes. The mean age of onset is 45 years; however, the earliest clinical manifestation is of migraine with aura which may occur before the age of 20 years. MRI is abnormal in all symptomatic patients and is characterized by absence of cortical lesions and hyperintense T2 signal changes of the periventricular and subcortical white matter, basal ganglia and pons. Small subcortical infarcts can be identified on T1-weighted images. MRI abnormalities can also be detected in pre-symptomatic family members. The condition is characterized by a typical arteriopathy with electron dense granular deposits in the media of the small cerebral arteries. The disease is due to mutations of the *Notch3* gene on chromosome 19. The condition shows an autosomal dominant pattern of inheritance with complete penetrance by the age of about 40 years. The mean age of death is 65 years.

144 i. The man has chemosis (conjunctival edema) and axial proptosis (**144a**). The diagnosis is traumatic carotico-cavernous fistula.
ii. There may be arterialized ('corkscrew') episcleral vessels, an orbital bruit, and sensory loss in the area of distribution of the ophthalmic division of the trigeminal nerve.
iii. The risks to vision are from retinal ischemia due to reduced arterio-venous perfusion gradient, glaucoma due to raised episcleral venous pressure, and corneal exposure due to proptosis.
iv. CT scanning or MRI will demonstrate the proptosis, enlarged extra-ocular muscles and

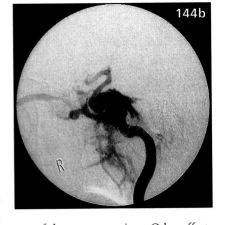

144b

superior ophthalmic vein, and possibly enlargement of the cavernous sinus. Other effects of the trauma may also be apparent, a basal skull fracture being particularly likely. The definitive investigation is carotid angiography. It is important to note that the clinical signs do not necessarily indicate the side of the fistula and four vessel angiography should be undertaken. In traumatic carotico-cavernous fistula, there is usually a large, direct fistula, i.e. communicating directly between the ICA and the cavernous sinus (**144b**). They are high flow and rarely close spontaneously. Balloon or coil embolization is the treatment of choice. Spontaneous carotico-cavernous fistulas tend to occur in older patients with diabetes mellitus or systemic hypertension. They are usually indirect, low-flow fistulas and commonly close spontaneously.

145 The 'locked-in' syndrome describes a state of:
(a) Prolonged coma.
(b) Bibrachial paresis with preserved leg movement.
(c) Severe spasticity after stroke.
(d) Quadriplegia with preserved vertical eye movements.

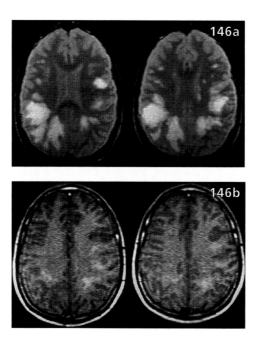

146 A 63-year-old, previously well female developed flu-like symptoms with pyrexia. She recovered completely from this but 2 weeks later she began to develop inco-ordination of her limbs and slurred speech, which evolved over several days. Her symptoms continued to progress and at the end of 1 week she had developed emotional lability and right upper and lower limb weakness. On examination she had a scanning dysarthria with broad-based gait. There was evidence of pyramidal weakness of the right arm and leg. CSF analysis performed after imaging revealed 56 lymphocytes/mm³. Protein was elevated at 1.45 g/L (0.145 g/dl). IgG oligoclonal bands were present in CSF but not in serum. A repeat CSF analysis 2 weeks later showed 40 lymphocytes/mm³ but no detectable oligoclonal bands. The MRI scans are a T2-weighted axial sequence (**146a**) and a T1-weighted coronal sequence (**146b**) after administration of gadolinium.
i. What does the MRI scan show?
ii. What is the most likely neurologic diagnosis in this patient?
iii. What treatment do you suggest?

145 (d) Quadriplegia with preserved vertical eye movements. The 'locked-in' syndrome describes a condition in which severe paralysis prevents any way of communicating except for preserved vertical eye movements, occasional blinking and eyelid closure. These patients are *not* comatose and often times are fully awake. Nearly all cases are due to basilar artery occlusion with extensive destruction of the basis pons, although isolated reports of midbrain lesions, traumatic brainstem injury, or spontaneous brainstem or cerebellar hemorrhages resulting in the locked-in syndrome do exist. The substrate for this condition is destruction of corticobulbar and corticospinal tracts with preservation of PPRF, leaving consciousness and vertical eye movements spared.

Bibrachial paresis describes the 'man-in-the-barrel' syndrome that often occurs after cardiac arrest and appears to be secondary to border zone ischemia in the territories between the middle and anterior cerebral arteries.

146 i. The MRI scan shows several confluent high signal lesions within white matter. The T1-weighted images demonstrate patchy enhancement within the lesions following administration of gadolinium – a paramagnetic contrast agent.
ii. This patient has had a monophasic inflammatory illness affecting several areas of the nervous system. The most likely diagnosis is an ADEM. The features that support this diagnosis are: (1) preceding infectious illness; (2) monophasic illness with no previous neurologic episodes; (3) intrathecal synthesis of IgG oligoclonal bands which then resolve; (4) enhancement of all lesions on MRI suggesting that they have developed simultaneously.

ADEM is an acute demyelinating disease, distinguished pathologically by numerous foci of inflammation and demyelination scattered throughout the brain and spinal cord. The foci surround small and medium sized veins. Axons are generally preserved. The disease usually follows a viral infection. A similar illness can occur following vaccination – particularly against rabies and very rarely after tetanus anti-toxin administration. The infectious agents most frequently associated with ADEM include Epstein–Barr virus, CMV, *Mycoplasma pneumoniae*, influenza, mumps, and HIV.

In terms of pathogenesis, the disease probably arises as a result of T-cell mediated immune reaction to components of myelin membrane or oligodendrocyte. Differential diagnosis includes a first demyelinating episode of MS, a viral meningo-encephalitis or a cerebral vasculitis.
iii. Treatment with i.v. methyl prednisolone 1 g for 3 days often speeds resolution of symptoms and signs by restoring the integrity of the blood–brain barrier. There have been some anecdotal reports of benefit from i.v. Ig in those patients who continue to progress despite steroid treatment, though this remains to be validated in a formal trial.

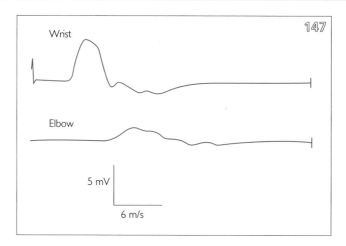

Wrist

Elbow

5 mV

6 m/s

147

147 A 43-year-old male was investigated for progressive weakness of left elbow flexion over the previous 2 years. He also noticed intermittent brief 'locking' of the fingers of the left hand over this time. CMAP tracings from the APB muscle are displayed, following supramaximal stimulation of the right median nerve at the wrist and elbow (147). The motor conduction velocity between these sites was 45 m/s. Similar findings were evident in the forearm segment of the left ulnar nerve and in the left tibial nerve. Normal sensory nerve conduction studies were obtained.
i. What neurophysiologic phenomenon is demonstrated?
ii. What is the likely diagnosis?

148 i. What two abnormal features can be seen in this patient (148)?
ii. What is the most likely cause of the rash?
iii. How would you treat this condition and the possible sequelae?

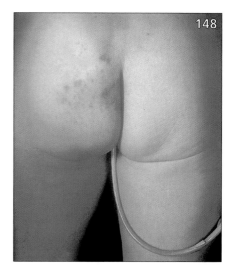

148

147 i. There is significant partial motor conduction block in the forearm segment of the right median nerve.
ii. The other findings indicate other sites of motor conduction block without sensory conduction abnormalities. This indicates multifocal motor conduction block. The locking symptom may be due to spontaneous muscle contractions after voluntary activation, resulting in failed or delayed relaxation of the relevant muscles. This may arise due to a region of hyperexcitability on the nerve. Some patients may have anti-GM1 antibodies detectable in serum, and would be expected to respond to i.v. immunoglobulin treatment.

148 i. Erythematous vesicular rash in a semicircular pattern over the medial aspect of the left buttock and urinary catheter.
ii. Varicella zoster infection/shingles. This is an unusual distribution for this viral condition, which occurs in a dermatomal distribution. It is most commonly seen unilaterally in the thoracic area, less frequently in the cervical area or involving the ophthalmic division of the trigeminal nerve, and rarely in the lumbosacral region, as in this case (left S3, S4, S5). The incidence is 3–5 per 1000 but increases with age and immunocompromised status. It is an extremely painful condition and up to 20% of patients develop post-herpetic neuralgia, a debilitating pain syndrome that persists after the rash has settled.
iii. The major goals of treatment are to relieve local discomfort, prevent dissemination in the immunocompromised individual, and prevent post-herpetic neuralgia. Various topical lotions, such as calamine, can partially ease the discomfort of the acute infection. The anti-viral drug, aciclovir, is active against the varicella zoster herpes virus but does not eradicate it. It is effective only if started at the onset of infection, and acts to reduce the duration of viral shedding and new lesion formation, speeds healing and lessens the acute pain. However, it is essential in the immunocompromised to try and reduce dissemination. If post-herpetic neuralgia does develop, amitryptiline or gabapentin, and occasionally carbamazepine or sodium valproate may improve control of the pain.

149 The angiogram shown here (149) was performed following unexplained hemiparesis in a 27-year-old female following a fall while rock climbing, in which she suffered a mild head injury, multiple facial fractures and a non-displaced cervical facet fracture. Examination of her pupils showed a right small pupil and ptosis.
i. What does the angiogram show?
ii. How often are vascular injuries associated with head injuries?

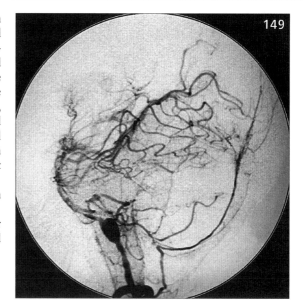

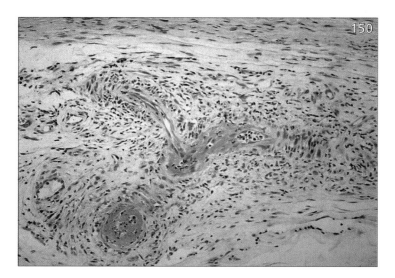

150 This is a nerve biopsy of a 30-year-old female with a 2-month history of mononeuritis multiplex (150). She was otherwise well.
What is shown in this nerve biopsy and what is the most likely diagnosis?

149 i. The angiogram demonstrates an ICA dissection.
ii. Previously, blunt traumatic vascular injuries were thought to be extremely rare. With screening, however, the incidence may be as high as 1% of blunt injuries. Mandible fractures, facial fractures, spine fractures and DAI appear to be associated with an increased incidence of blunt vascular injury. A high index of suspicion must be maintained as sequelae are often delayed in presentation with disastrous, irreversible consequences.

150 This nerve biopsy shows necrotizing vasculitis of an arteriole. There is a dense mononuclear inflammatory cell infiltrate, fibrinoid necrosis of the intima, and narrowing of the lumen with intraluminal thrombosis. These are the features seen in vasculitis. Conditions including polyarteritis nodosa, Churg–Strauss syndrome, Behçet's syndrome, connective tissue diseases, Sjögren's syndrome, sarcoidosis, Wegener's granulomatosis, cryoglobulinemia, and HIV infection need to be considered. If the patient has no evidence of vasculitis elsewhere the diagnosis is likely to be nerve specific vasculitis. The ESR may be elevated in this condition but is often normal. Patients usually present with a mononeuritis multiplex, but they may present with a symmetric sensory and motor neuropathy. Pain may be a feature and is a clue to the diagnosis. Nerve conduction studies usually confirm a mononeuritis multiplex and may be particularly useful in patients with a symmetric neuropathy clinically because they may suggest that the neuropathy is patchy or asymmetric. Nerve biopsy is usually needed to make the diagnosis but the yield is higher if a combined nerve and muscle biopsy is performed.

Treatment is not always necessary in nerve specific vasculitis as the condition has a better prognosis than systemic vasculitis. However, if the neuropathy is causing significant morbidity (especially pain or motor deficit) then treatment should be given. Treatment is usually with steroids and patients sometimes respond to lower doses than systemic vasculitis patients. Azathioprine may be needed as a steroid sparing agent and cyclophosphamide may be needed in the more severe cases if further immunosuppression is required. In one large series, about one-third of cases recovered; about one-quarter of cases relapsed when treatment was stopped; and about one-third of cases progressed to develop systemic vasculitis with a consequently worse prognosis.

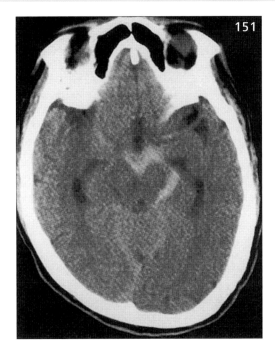

151 This 51-year-old female presents with grade I SAH and this CT scan (**151**). Her angiogram is entirely unremarkable.
i. What is the likely diagnosis?
ii. What further work-up would you recommend?

152 A 20-year-old female first presented with seizures at the age of 18 years. These were of generalized tonic–clonic type. She also complained of brief episodes lasting minutes of experiencing blobs of color masking her vision. In addition, she reported separate episodes of 'jumpiness' of her arms and legs with preserved consciousness. There was no family history of neurologic diseases, although she was born of consanguineous parents. Despite treatment with phenytoin, the seizures worsened and she developed severe flurries of brief random jerks in all four limbs. Two years later, she has continued to deteriorate, with child-like regression and global cognitive decline. On examination, she is deaf and her speech interrupted by choreiform mouth movements. Noises and reflex testing provoke flurries of severe jerking occurring in random patterns separately in all limbs.
i. Was her initial treatment appropriate?
ii. Into what subgroup would her jerking disorder be classified?
iii. What is the likely diagnosis?

151

151 i. Perimesencephalic SAH, the etiology of which is unknown.
ii. Given the perfect angiogram, the classic CT image with no extension of blood into the sylvian or interhemispheric fissures, and her good clinical grade, many experts now recommend no further work-up. Certainly, given these findings a single follow-up angiogram at 2 weeks suffices. If there is any focal spasm, the CT is not classic, there is an atypical blood pattern or she is grade III or worse, the diagnosis should be doubted and early and late (1 month) angiography should be undertaken. It should also be noted that angiography should include the EC system to rule out a dural AVF, and a high spinal and brain MRI should be performed to rule out spinal AVM/AVF and other strange variants. A detailed coagulation work-up should also be undertaken.

152 i. No. As well as generalized seizures, her experience of colored blobs in her vision were likely to represent simple focal occipital seizures. Her jerky movements were likely to be myoclonic in type. Myoclonus may be defined as a brief, sometimes as little as 30 ms, contraction of a muscle or group of muscles resulting in a body jerk. It may be repetitive, but is distinguished from tremor on the basis that the movement is unidirectional rather than bidirectional. Phenytoin is not a very effective anti-convulsant for simple partial seizure and may in fact worsen myoclonus. Better choices would have been sodium valproate, lamotrigine or perhaps topiramate. The myoclonic jerks may themselves have been treated with clonazepam and piracetam.
ii. Myclonus may be classified according to the likely location of origin or according to etiology. A random pattern of jerking in different limbs with a focal stimulus sensitivity is suggestive of cortical myoclonus. An etiologic classification of myoclonus might include physiologic myoclonus (e.g. hypnopompic jerks), essential myoclonus (idiopathic and occurring in isolation), epileptic myoclonus (part of a characteristic and generally non-progressive epileptic syndrome), progressive myoclonic epilepsy, progressive myoclonic ataxia (progressive inherited diseases with the characteristic combination of features), and symptomatic myoclonus (other underlying structural diseases, focal lesions or encephalopathies).

This patient's initial presentation with epilepsy and myoclonus and subsequent severe generalized deterioration, together with her susceptibility to recessively inherited disease, would make it most likely that she has a progressive myoclonic epilepsy.
iii. Lafora body disease. The autosomal recessive progressive myoclonic epilepsy presents usually in late adolescence or early childhood. Characteristic features are the severe stimulus sensitive myoclonic flurries, behavioral problems, simple visual hallucinations and deafness later on. The disease is relentlessly progressive. It is a storage disease and may be diagnosed from an axilla skin biopsy by polyglycosan accumulation in the duct cells of eccrine sweat glands. It relates to a mutation of *protein tyrosine phosphatase* gene on chromosome 6.

153 A 15-year-old female with cognitive decline for the last 3 years has on examination mild dystonia of her arms and vertical gaze palsy. The figure shows an electron microscopy of a bone marrow histiocyte (153). Her family history is negative.
i. What is the likely diagnosis?
ii. What is the inheritance?
iii. Is there a laboratory method for confirming the diagnosis?

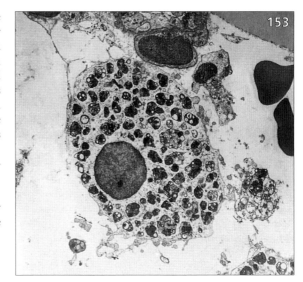

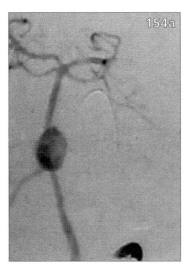
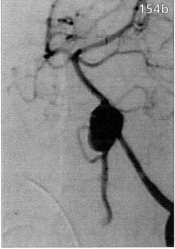

154 This 34-year-old female presents with a SAH.
i. What do the angiograms show (154a, b)?
ii. What surgical approaches can be considered for this lesion?
iii. How can the vertebral artery be identified as it enters the dura?

153 i. The likely diagnosis is NPD type C. This is a neurometabolic disorder characterized by cognitive and behavioral decline with vertical supranuclear ophthalmoplegia and ataxia. Involuntary movements, seizures and pyramidal signs are other later features. Hepatosplenomegaly is present, but less severe than in NPD types A and B. NPD type A is a severe infantile neurogenetic disorder with hepato-splenomegaly. NPD type B has no neurologic involvement, a later onset of hepato-splenomegaly and survival into adulthood.

ii. The inheritance pattern for NPD type C is autosomal recessive.

iii. The biochemical defect is an abnormality in cholesterol transport, leading to the accumulation of sphingomyelin and cholesterol in lysosomes. The laboratory method for confirmation of NPD type C is measuring intracellular cholesterol esterification and filipin staining of free cholesterol in cultured skin fibroblasts. This testing is commercially available and confirms the clinical diagnosis of NPD type C. NPD types A and B are diagnosed by marked sphingomyelinase deficiency, which is normal in type C. The bone marrow in types A, B and C show the characteristic lipid laden phagocytic foam cells or Niemann–Pick cells.

154 i. The angiogram shows a vertebro-basilar junction aneurysm.

ii. Surgical approaches to this lesion include: (1) ELITE approach; (2) a combined retrosigmoid and presigmoid petrosal approach; or (3) retrolabyrinthine, trans-sigmoid approach. These approaches move the point of entry to the posterior fossa forward; as the entry point to the posterior fossa approaches the plane of the clivus retraction of the cerebellum and brainstem is reduced and depth of dissection increased. The ELITE approach alters the trajectory to pathologies anterior to the lower brainstem from a posterior orientation to a more lateral–inferior approach. If the vertebro-basilar junction is in a very high location, then a petrosal approach may be required. Approaches such as a subtemporal transtentorial or transcavernous approach are generally suited to lesions arising from the middle third of the basilar artery up. A combined supratentorial and intratentorial approach is useful for lesions between the vertebro-basilar junction and the AICA. A lateral suboccipital approach is suitable for VA–PICA aneurysms.

iii. The VA turns anterolaterally around the lateral mass of C1 just before it enters the dura. Between C1 and C2 a vertebral venous plexus warns the surgeon that the VA is nearby. The dorsal ramus of C2 runs posterior to the VA and C1 and C2 and can serve as a guide to the artery.

155 A 70-year-old male with hypertension and diabetes is seen in the emergency department. On examination, he is comatose with reactive pupils. Laboratory data are as follows: Na^+ = 118 mmol/L (mEq/L), K^+ = 3.8 mmol/L (mEq/L), HCO_3^- = 27 mmol/L (mEq/L), urea 9 mmol/L (BUN 25 mg/dl), creatinine 186 µmol/L (2.1 mg/dl), glucose 14 mmol/L (252 mg/dl). Blood pressure is 120/80 mmHg (16/10.7 kPa).
i. Which of the following is the likely cause of the patient's comatose state?
(a) Uremia.
(b) Stroke.
(c) Hyponatremia.
(d) DKA.
ii. What is the best treatment for the above condition?
(a) Dialysis.
(b)Thrombolysis.
(c) Salt tablets.
(d) Fluid restriction.

156 A 35-year-old male presented with an acute confusional state. On admission the Glasgow coma scale was 15, temperature 38.6°C (101.5°F). He gradually became obtunded and required ventilation.
i. What abnormalities are evident on the CT scan (**156**)?
ii. What other tests are indicated?
iii. What is the treatment?

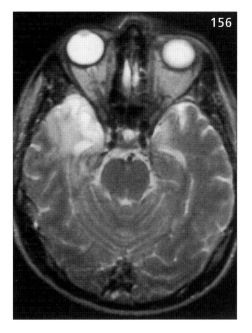

155 i. (c). Depressed levels of consciousness usually occur when serum sodium levels fall below 125; seizures are more frequent below levels of 120. The reactive pupils on examination suggest lack of structural cause (e.g. stroke, tumor) for the coma. Evaluation of hyponatremia includes assessment of volume status as either hyper-, hypo-, or normovolemic. Important laboratory values to be obtained include urine sodium and chloride concentrations, and serum and urine osmolality. Urine sodium concentrations <20 mmol/L (mEq/L) usually indicates hypovolemia, while increased urine sodium >20 mmol/L (mEq/L) is seen in cerebral salt wasting, patients with metabolic alkalosis from profuse vomiting, and the syndrome of SIADH. Other causes of hyponatremia with hypovolemia include diuretics and Addison's disease; with normo- or hypervolemia include acute renal or hepatic failure, congestive heart failure, and SIADH. Correction of severe hyponatremia in cases of SIADH should be undertaken slowly and cautiously, i.e. the rate of correction should not be >12–15 mmol/L (mEq/L) over the first 24 hours. A more rapid correction could result in the development of central or extrapontine myelinolysis with demyelination in the basis pontis, cerebellum, putamen, thalamus, or subcortical white matter tracts. Maintenance fluids with i.v. normal saline are recommended and avoidance of hypotonic solutions, such as dextrose saline or one-half normal saline, the rule.
ii. (d). Usually, fluid restriction can correct even a severe hyponatremic state. Occasionally, refractory hyponatremia can be corrected by giving 3% saline at a slow rate calculated as the total sodium deficit to be corrected at a specified desired correction rate (0.5 mmol/L/hour [mEq/L/hour]). Frequent, periodic determination of serum sodium levels are necessary to guide therapy.

156 i. There is generalized brain swelling with low density change in the right temporal lobe. In view of the swelling a lumbar puncture was contraindicated. One was performed 3 weeks later and this showed 17 lymphocytes/mm³, protein 2.43 mg/L (0.243 mg/dl), sugar 4.2 mmol/L (75.7 mg/dl) with a blood sugar of 5.6 mmol/L (100.9 mg/dl). PCR for herpes simplex was negative which is not surprising given the delay.
ii. EEG. The distinctive pattern in herpes simplex encephalitis consists of periodic slow- and sharp-wave wave complexes occurring every 2–3 seconds. They may occur uni- or bilaterally.
iii. Herpes simplex virus type 1 is the most common cause of sporadic encephalitis in adults. In the immunosuppressed patient herpes varicella-zoster, Epstein–Barr virus and CMV may all cause an encephalitic illness. In this patient where lumbar puncture was not safe, an important differential is a bacterial meningitis with an area of cerebritis or early abscess formation. Treatment should be i.v. aciclovir and it would be prudent to cover the possibility of a bacterial infection with a third generation cephalosporin antibiotic such as ceftriaxone.

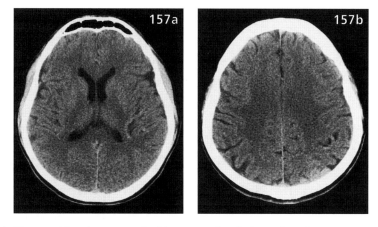

157 A 41-year-old male presented with a severe headache and a seizure.
i. What does the nonenhanced CT (157a, b) show?
ii. What is the likely diagnosis based on these findings?
iii. What study would you order to further evaluate this patient?

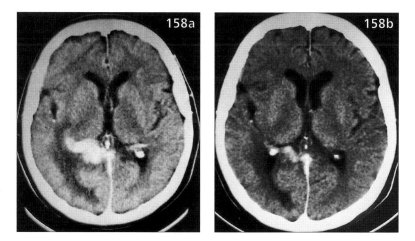

158 A 79-year-old female was admitted to hospital with a 3-week history of intermittent confusion. She was systemically well and apyrexial. There was no focal neurology. An infection screen was negative. A CT scan was performed (158a), she was given some tablets and the CT scan repeated 4 days later (158b) after considerable improvement.
i. What is the likely diagnosis?
ii. What treatment was she given?

157 i. The nonenhanced CT shows subtle enlargement of several left MCA branches (**157c**, arrows) and parietal veins (**157d**, arrow).
ii. The nonenhanced CT findings are definitely abnormal and suggest a small left parietal AVM. While AVMs can be invisible on nonenhanced CT scans, asymmetrically enlarged arteries and veins are a valuable clue to their presence.
iii. The next study should be either a contrast enhanced CT scan or an MRI examination, both of which can exclude all but the smallest AVMs. In this case, a

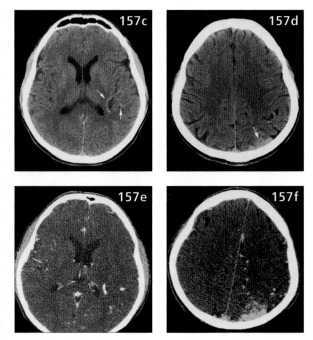

thin section helical CT scan was obtained during the arterial phase of contrast infusion and confirmed a left parietal AVM with MCA supply and cortical venous drainage (**157e, f**). Helical scanning permits rapid acquisition of CT slices during the short period of time when an i.v. infusion of iodinated contrast opacifies intracerebral arteries. Infusion CT scanning, also called CTA, is useful for identifying vascular malformations and aneurysms in the setting of intracerebral, subarachnoid, or intraventricular hemorrhage.

158 i. Primary CNS lymphoma.
ii. Steroids (dexamethasone). The scan and response to steroids is typical of PCNSL. This tumor is rare but steadily increasing in incidence, even without the AIDS epidemic. It is essentially a local disease with <10% of patients having evidence of systemic disease at autopsy. Many lesions are periventricular, which predisposes to dissemination through the CSF. There is usually intense and homogeneous contrast enhancement on CT scanning. PCNSL is exquisitely sensitive to the lympholytic effects of steroids and so they should not be started before diagnostic biopsy. The treatment of this condition is based around high dose MTX chemotherapy followed by radiotherapy. Unlike systemic lymphoma, the conventional CHOP regimen provides only short-lived benefit.

159 A 30-year-old male i.v. drug user felt feverish and unwell a few hours after injecting himself with heroin. Twenty-four hours later he complained of head and neck ache. Examination showed a mild spastic quadriplegia, more evident in the legs than the arms. There was a sensory level to pinprick to C3–C4.
i. What is the likely diagnosis?
ii. What is the most likely organism?
iii. What other blood and imaging studies may be necessary?

160 A 22-year-old, right-handed female is referred for the futher management of her epilepsy. She had a prolonged febrile convulsion in infancy. She has frequent complex partial seizures with an aura of fear and a rising epigastric sensation followed by impairment of consciousness. Witnesses describe how she may utter simple phrases during seizures, will fiddle with her right hand, and be confused after attacks, on one occasion burning herself on her gas cooker. She has never had secondarily generalized seizures, but her complex partial seizures have not responded to treatment with phenytoin, valproate, carbamazepine, lamotrigine or topiramate. Her attacks tend to cluster around menses.

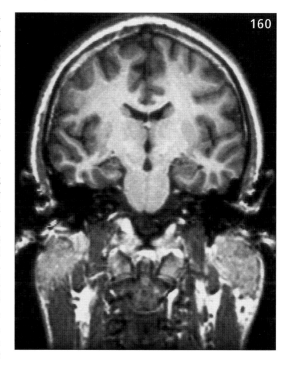

160

i. What does the MRI scan show (**160**)?
ii. What is your management strategy?

159 i. Spinal epidural abscess (159a, b, arrows).
ii. The commonest organism causing epidural abscesses is *Staphylococcus aureus*. Other pathogens include Gram negative bacilli, *Streptococcus pneumoniae*, and *Staphylococcus epidermididis*. In areas of the world where there is a high prevalence, *Mycobacteria tuberculosis* is a relatively frequent cause.
iii. Blood cultures may isolate the causative organism. In an i.v. drug user, endocarditis may be a complication and i.v. drug users are at risk of developing HIV Infection.

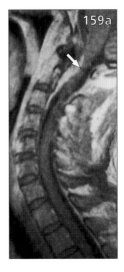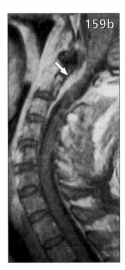

160 i. The MRI shows loss of volume of the right hippocampus. In this setting, the cause is almost invariably hippocampal sclerosis. This could be further substantiated on T2-weighted or proton-density sequences, which might also show increased signal in the right mesial temporal region.
ii. The history is typical of refractory temporal lobe epilepsy due to hippocampal sclerosis, associated with an early prolonged febrile convulsion. Her seizure semiology would be typical for a right temporal lobe seizure in a right-handed individual. The resistance to drug treatment is common in epilepsy due to hippocampal sclerosis (90% of cases are refractory to medical treatment). Her epilepsy is clearly serious – she has burnt herself already. Though she may not have an increased risk of sudden death, in the absence of secondarily generalized seizures and not being male, nevertheless she is at increased risk of morbidity and requires careful counseling about lifestyle issues. She is a potential surgical candidate. She requires referral to an epilepsy center, where she is likely to have at least videotelemetry, which is the first step in determining her suitability for surgery and prognosis therefrom. She may have up to a 70–80% chance at best of becoming seizure free. In the meantime, if there is a true catamenial predominance to seizures, the option of perimenstrual clobazam therapy (e.g. 10 mg/day for 7 days around her menses) would be worth considering, in addition to the option of altering her prophylactic anti-epileptic drugs. As for all women of child-bearing age, the issues of contraception and teratogenicity must be discussed if this has not already been undertaken.

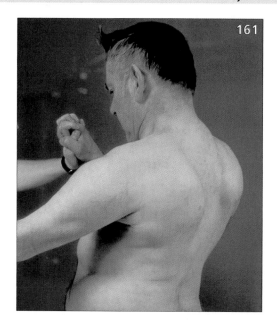

161 This patient's findings are winging of the scapula (**161**), mild facial weakness and pectoral muscle atrophy. His father has never been able to whistle and the paternal grandmother is in a wheelchair.
i. What is the diagnosis?
ii. What is the inheritance pattern?
iii. How does this family demonstrate variable expressivity of a genetic disease?
iv. Is there a DNA test available?

162 A 70-year-old male initially presented with unsteadiness of gait and stiffness of the limbs. He was given treatment and the stiffness improved but he then developed behavioral problems and visual hallucinations. Despite reduction in this medication and introduction of new medication his condition continues to deteriorate in a fluctuating manner with worsening rigidity: on some days he is rather active, especially at night, while on others he remains in bed markedly rigid and virtually comatose. Examination reveals a severe bradyphrenia and cognitive defect when able to co-operate. He has dysphagia and marked dysarthria, rigid limbs with brisk reflexes and upgoing plantar responses. He displays myoclonic jerks of the limbs.
i. What is the diagnosis?
ii. What type of medication was he first given?
iii. What was he given next?

161 i. The patient has FSHD. It is suspected in the presence of muscular weakness of the face, scapular fixator, proximal arm, and hip girdle. Disease onset is usually in the teens, but is highly variable.

ii. It is inherited in an autosomal dominant manner. Offspring of affected individuals have a 50% chance of inheriting the gene for FSHD.

iii. Expressivity is the range of clinical characteristics of a genetic disorder. Variable expressivity means that the disease may show a wide range of clinical phenotypes from mild to severe in individuals who have the disease mutation. FSHD is a well-recognized example of variable expressivity. The disease varies in severity and age of onset even in the same family. The severity may vary from individuals requiring a wheelchair to mild problems such as facial weakness or no symptoms at all. More than 90% of the affected individuals show findings by the age of 20 years.

iv. Genetic testing is available. It is not a direct gene mutation assay. The gene for FSHD is not known, but it is linked to chromosome 4q35. The test detects micro-deletions of DNA in that region. The test is generally accurate, but should be interpreted in conjunction with the clinical picture.

162 i. Dementia with Lewy bodies. This is a variant of parkinsonism in which, unlike idiopathic Parkinson's disease where Lewy body abnormalities are mainly restricted to the substantia nigra compacta of the midbrain, there are also widespread Lewy bodies in the cerebral cortex and other structures, such as areas CA2 and 3 of the hippocampus. The condition may present with an akinetic-rigid syndrome or there may be a more psychiatric presentation with confusion, behavioral problems (such as reversal of the day–night activity cycle), and complex, often rather banal, visual hallucinations. Early on, patients may tend to suffer frequent falls, while later in the disease's course there may be rather dramatic fluctuations in consciousness. There may be myoclonus, tremor and pyramidal signs. The prognosis is worse than in idiopathic Parkinson's disease.

ii. The patient was given levodopa to alleviate the bradykinesia and rigidity. Unfortunately, in dementia with Lewy bodies, while the akinetic-rigid features may respond to such medication, there may be extreme sensitivity to psychiatric side effects. This is often how the true diagnosis becomes apparent.

iii. Conversely, patients also display neuroleptic sensitivity so that small doses of a neuroleptic for hallucinations or night-time disturbance result in severe akinesia and rigidity. As many patients initially present with such features, dementia with Lewy bodies is often diagnosed on the basis of this reaction.

When attempting to treat this condition, a neuroleptic with minimal extra-pyramidal side effects is selected, such as sulpiride, olanzapine or sertindole. Patients may be able to tolerate a small dose of levodopa or anticholinergic for their rigidity. In dementia with Lewy bodies, there may be a favorable response to the CNS anti-cholinesterase inhibitors donepezil and rivastigmine, perhaps better than in AD.

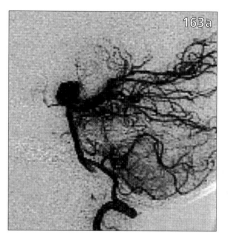
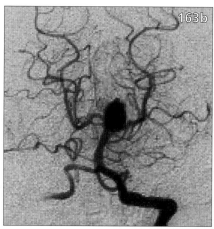

163 This 51-year-old female presents with grade I SAH and this basilar apex aneurysm (163a, b).
i. What are the pros and cons to GDC?
ii. What are the pros and cons to surgery?
iii. How would you manage it?

164 A 52-year-old female with relapsed stage IVB non-Hodgkin's lymphoma was treated with a stem cell transplant 2 months ago. She then developed focal seizures and a weakness of her left arm and increasing lethargy. She was apyrexial and did not complain of headache. A CT brain scan was performed (164).
i. What is the differential diagnosis?
ii. What are the principles of management?

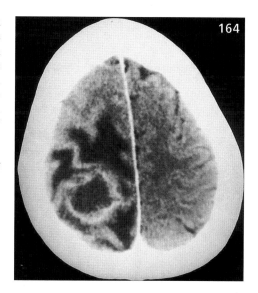

163 i. GDC of basilar apex aneurysms has a lower procedural complication rate in most centers than clipping. In addition the basilar apex is a 'straight shot' for coil deployment. Recurrence at this location is, however, quite common especially with wide-necked aneurysms such as this one. Balloon remodeling techniques and 3D coils may be improving matters but still this neck is less than ideal.

ii. Except at centers with vast experience this is a very dangerous lesion, given its height above the clinoids and its projection back into the brainstem which makes preservation of the perforators difficult. Nonetheless with orbitozygomatic craniotomy, temporary vessel occlusion and fenestrated clips this can be clipped with lasting surgical cure.

iii. There is no right answer other than it needs to be treated. Two additional options are: (1) to explore the aneurysm for clipping and backout if the perforators are not easy to free (in such a case coiling would be performed immediately); (2) subtotal coiling followed by delayed exploration after the vasospasm risk has passed. In either case protection of the dome should be the first priority and delay should be minimized in this intact patient.

164 i. The scan shows a ring-enhanced mass lesion in her right frontoparietal lobe with surrounding edema. The radiologic differential diagnosis is wide but in the context of an immunosuppressed patient the most likely differentials include fungal abscess, cerebral toxoplasmosis, nocardia and bacterial abscess. Intracerebral metastases from non-Hodgkin's lymphoma are extremely rare.

ii. Broad spectrum anti-bacterial, anti-fungal and anti-protozoal cover. Do a biopsy if no improvement is observed within 1 week to guide further treatment. Perform aspiration and surgical decompression if there are symptoms and signs of rising ICP. CNS infections are an uncommon complication of cancer and are usually seen in patients with lymphoma and leukemia, often after chemotherapy and bone marrow transplantation. The usual florid symptoms apparent in immunocompetent patients with CNS infection are not seen in these patients. In particular, headache and fever may be absent (as in this patient). Brain abscesses are usually due to fungi, nocardia or toxoplasma, i.e. a different group of pathogens compared to immuncompetent patients, and need to be covered with appropriate antibiotics. Surgical intervention should be reserved when the conscious level declines or when there is no improvement after 1 week of appropriate treatment. Often other foci of infection, e.g. lung abscesses due to nocardia, allow precise diagnosis without the need for a brain biopsy.

165 A 24-year-old female gave a 2-day history of headache. She had developed a severe generalized throbbing headache, accompanied by photophobia, nausea, vomiting, and mild left-sided weakness which had persisted since onset and was subsequently confirmed on examination. There was no past history of headache but her mother suffered from migraine with aura. She was 1 week post-partum and had had a vaginal delivery without complication.

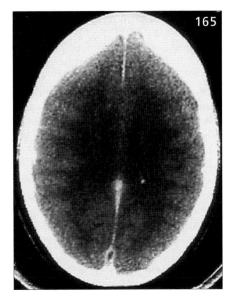

i. What are the two main differential diagnoses in this patient?
ii. What investigation has been performed (165)?
iii. What does it show?

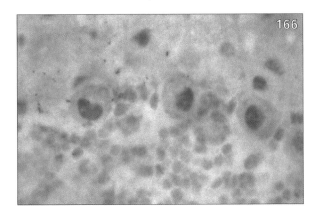

166 A 56-year-old female presented with a 5-month history of paresthesias and numbness in her feet. On examination she was areflexic and had severely diminished proprioception to her knees and wrists. Nerve conduction studies showed a sensory axonal polyneuropathy. A chest X-ray revealed a small shadow behind the right hilum. This is a histological slide of human cerebellum stained with the patient's serum (166).
i. What special blood test was requested and what does it show?
ii. What further investigation should be done to confirm this test?

165 i. The two main differential diagnoses are of a first episode of migraine with aura (since the duration is greater than 60 minutes, the aura symptoms are by definition prolonged), and of cerebral venous sinus thrombosis.
ii. A CT head scan with contrast has been performed.
iii. The imaging shows isodense clot in the sagittal sinus, the 'delta sign', indicative of sagittal sinus thrombosis. Post-partum headache occurs in about 40% of women most frequently in the first week, and is common in individuals with a history or family history of migraine. About 60% of migraineurs will develop headache post-partum. Migraine tends to improve during pregnancy, usually in the second and third trimester, but can occur for the first time in pregnancy more commonly during the first trimester. Cerebral venous thrombosis occurs more frequently in pregnancy and the puerperium. Although migraine can occur for the first time during the puerperium, cerebral venous thrombosis should be considered in this patient presenting with new onset persistent headache and focal neurology. No cause is usually found. However, the patient should be investigated to look for a predisposition to thromboembolism.

166 i. Anti-neuronal antibodies. This section of human cerebellum shows the presence of anti-neuronal antibodies, which stain upon all the neuronal nuclei and the cytoplasm to a lesser extent.
ii. Western blotting against either recombinant Hu antigen or a cerebellar preparation looking for bands at 35–40 kD. This would confirm that the patient had anti-Hu antibodies, which are found in paraneoplastic neuropathies particularly associated with small cell lung cancer. Other neurologic syndromes associated with these antibodies include paraneoplastic encephalomyelitis/sensory neuropathy. The anti-Hu syndrome is the most common paraneoplastic syndrome affecting the CNS, and the presence of characteristic anti-neuronal antibodies guides the clinician to an otherwise asymptomatic malignancy. This patient was subsequently shown to have a small cell lung cancer. Interestingly, these antibodies are found in about 15% of neurologically normal patients with lung cancer and may be associated with a better oncologic prognosis.

Nerve conduction studies

Right	Lat (ms)	Amp (μV)	Vel m/s	F (ms)	Left	Lat (ms)	Amp (μV)	Vel m/s	F (ms)
Motor									
Median: wrist	3.7	5500		28.2		3.2	17 800		24.7
elbow		4800	59				15 000	59	
axilla		3900	56						
Ulnar: wrist	2.2	5700		28.0		1.8	10 800		25.8
below elbow		5000	50				8 500	53	
above elbow		5000	48						
Sensory									
Radial		28	63				25	63	
Median: digit I		53	66				30	69	
digit II		39	62				27	65	
digit III		14	60				22	64	
digit IV		2	55				17	62	
Ulnar: digit IV		3	61				13	67	
digit V		6	66				12	69	
Medial antebrachial		No response					22	61	
Lateral antebrachial		32	57				27	57	

167 These nerve conduction studies were recorded from a 26-year-old male with an 8-month history of progressive numbness over the medial aspect of the right hand and forearm, weakness in the right hand, and aching in the left upper arm (*see table*).
i. What are the main abnormalities?
ii. What is the diagnosis?
iii. What investigation should be carried out next?

168 This 50-year-old female presents with hearing loss. Speech discrimination score is 30% and the auditory threshold is 20 dB.
i. What does the MRI show (**168**)?
ii. Is hearing preservation a realistic goal in treating this lesion?
iii. What surgical approaches should be considered?
iv. Is gamma knife therapy an option?
v. When approaching this lesion from the posterior fossa what is the location of facial nerve in relation to the tumor in decreasing frequency of occurrence?

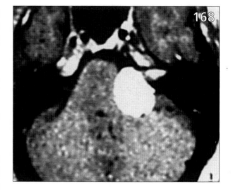

167 i. There is evidence of complete sensory axonal loss in the right medial antebrachial nerve, and of significant partial sensory axonal loss in the right ulnar nerve and in the right median nerve from digits III and IV. The low amplitude CMAPs from the right APB and ADM muscles are consistent with additional motor axonal loss in the nerves to these muscles.

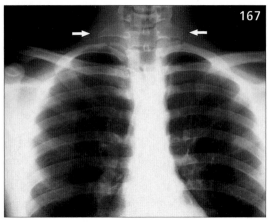

ii. These findings indicate a right-sided significant partial inferior brachial plexopathy, such as can occur with neurogenic thoracic outlet syndrome.

iii. A chest X-ray should be carried out, and may detect evidence of cervical ribs (167, arrows).

168 i. The patient has vestibular schwannoma.

ii. Hearing preservation is unlikely. Two factors predict whether functional hearing can be preserved: tumor size, and audiologic assessment. Useful hearing is unlikely if speech discrimination is <50%, auditory threshold is <50 dB, and when the tumor size is >2.5 cm (1 in) in diameter.

iii. Surgical approaches to this particular lesion include translabyrinthine, and retrosigmoid (suboccipital). If hearing preservation were a goal then a retrosigmoid suboccipital approach would be preferred. The middle fossa approach is not indicated in this lesion; it is best used for small intracanalicular lesions.

iv. Gamma knife is an option when tumor volume is <10 ml or diameter is <2.5–3 cm (1–1.2 in). Initial experience with gamma knife therapy using a dose of 20 Gy to the tumor periphery resulted in a very high incidence of cranial nerve palsies (80%). More recently, lower doses 11–14 Gy at the tumor periphery have been found to provide tumor control (90%) with a very low incidence of facial or trigeminal palsies (<5%). Hearing is unchanged in 30% of the patients but usually deteriorates in the remaining patients.

v. From a suboccipital approach, the facial nerve is found anterior to the tumor in about half the cases, superior in 30%, and inferior in 15%.

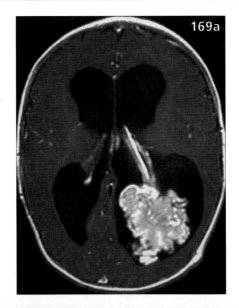

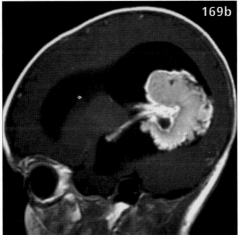

169 You are called to see a 3-month-old male with poor feeding, mild developmental delay, a head circumference greater than the 95% percentile, and a bulging anterior fontanelle. His brain MRI is shown (**169a, b**).

i. What is the most likely diagnosis?
ii. List two possible etiologies for his hydrocephalus.
iii. How would you treat this patient?
iv. What is the major differential diagnosis pathologically?

169 i. The most likely diagnosis is a choroid plexus tumor. The majority are benign (choroid plexus papilloma), although malignant tumors also occur (choroid plexus carcinomas). While in children these tumors occur primarily supratentorially in the lateral and third ventricles, most choroid plexus tumors arise infratentorially (fourth ventricle) in adults.

ii. Hydrocephalus principally occurs from the mass effect of the tumor with obstruction of the foramen of Monro. These tumors can also overproduce CSF and release protein, both known to increase the risk of hydrocephalus.

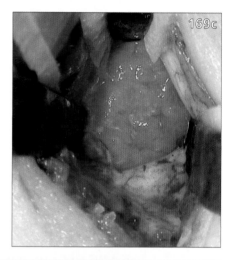

iii. Benign lesions can be cured surgically with total removal (**169c**), and even malignant tumors respond well to surgery. Complete resection can be difficult because of bleeding from the choroidal arteries and the fragility and size of the tumor (**169d**). Re-operation may be necessary if recurrence occurs. Hydrocephalus in some patients is not cured by resection of the tumor, and may require shunting.

iv. Pathologically, the major differential diagnosis is between a choroid plexus papilloma and a papillary ependymoma. Distinguishing characteristics are shown in the table below.

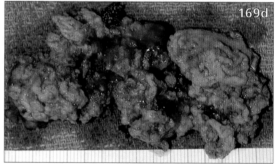

Distinguishing characteristics of choroid plexus papilloma and papillary ependymoma

	Choroid plexus papilloma/carcinoma	Papillary ependymoma
Architecture	Epithelial with fibrovascular stroma	Epithelial with glial stroma
Immunocytochemistry	Cytokeratin (+)	Cytokeratin (–)
	CEA (+) (carcinoma)	CEA (–)
	Prealbumin (+) (papilloma)	
Intraventricular location	Yes	Yes

170 A 45-year-old male was found unconscious with evidence of dried blood on his scalp. He was brought to the emergency department where he was intubated. He had elevated blood pressure, non-reactive pupils and extensor posturing. There were no other apparent injuries. A head CT was performed (170).
i. What does the head CT show?
ii. Are these types of injury always fatal?
iii. What is the appropriate treatment?

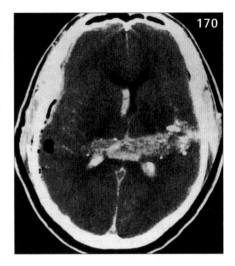

171 A 31-year-old female has a 20-year history of seizures in which she first has a feeling of fear that rises up from her stomach, and then she occasionally loses touch with her surroundings for approximately 10 minutes. During this period, she walks around as if in a dream and fiddles with her clothes, and after this she is confused for 5–10 minutes. These seizures are resistant to medication. The only past history of note was a series of seizures with fever in the first couple of years of life. An MRI was performed (171).
i. What type of seizures does she describe?
ii. What does the MRI show?
iii. What is the association between this pathology and her past medical history?

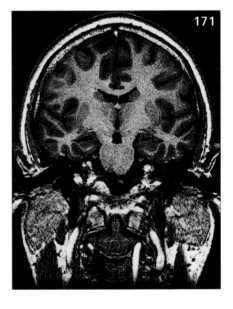

170 i. The head CT shows a transventricular GSW.

ii. Because transventricular GSWs usually involve the diencephalon or brainstem they are often fatal. Not all GSWs to the head are fatal, however. In fact, many result in injury of non-eloquent brain, allowing for a recovery with grossly normal function.

iii. If deemed non-fatal, a GSW to the head should be treated with a craniotomy. It is important to debride severely injured brain and irrigate the tract copiously to decrease the chance of infection. Dural defects should be repaired. This can be accomplished using pericranial patch grafts. Finally, in some cases it may be necessary to repair bone defects with split thickness bone autografts prior to debridement and closure of the skin. Post-operative antibiotics are often indicated.

171 i. Partial seizures in which consciousness is impaired are referred to as complex partial seizures. They may evolve from simple partial seizures (as in this instance), resulting in an aura, or may occur with impairment of consciousness at onset. The nature of the complex partial seizure is determined by the lobar origin. The seizure described is typical for a complex partial seizure originating in the temporal lobe. In temporal lobe seizures the aura commonly consists of: rising epigastric sensation, autonomic symptoms, psychic symptoms (especially *déjà vu*, depersonalization, memory flashbacks, fear, anger) or hallucinations (especially gustatory and olfactory). Automatisms commonly occur and consist of fumbling, picking clothes, lip smacking and chewing.

ii. The MRI demonstrates a smaller hippocampus on the right – typical for hippocampal sclerosis (mesial temporal sclerosis). The hippocampus is an archeo-cortical structure, in the medial part of the temporal lobe. It is part of the limbic system.

iii. Febrile convulsions are a common cause of hippocampal sclerosis. Febrile convulsions, however, are usually benign with only 7% of children with febrile convulsions developing epilepsy by the age of 25 years. The greatest risk of developing epilepsy is in those with a prolonged febrile convulsion (longer than 20 minutes), focal features in the convulsion, a family history of epilepsy (non-febrile convulsions), and prior abnormal neurology or development.

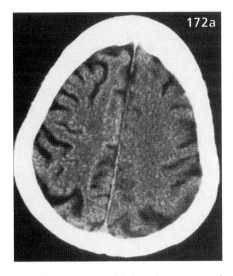

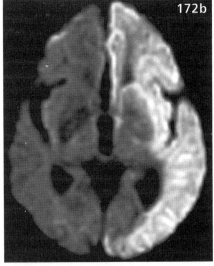

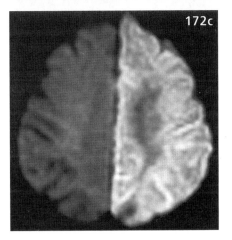

172 An 83-year-old female presented with acute right hemiparesis. A non-enhanced CT scan (172a) and diffusion MRI (172b, c) were obtained to confirm the clinical diagnosis of acute cerebral infarct.

i. Are there any abnormal findings on the nonenhanced CT?

ii. What is the vascular distribution of the infarct?

iii. What is the physiologic basis for the signal abnormalities on diffusion MRI? How soon after a cerebral infarct can they be detected? How long do they last?

173 The following could be used to control elevated ICP except:
(a) Mannitol 0.5–1.0 g/kg i.v.
(b) Head of bed elevation of 30°.
(c) Hyperventilation to pCO_2 of 28 mmHg (3.7 kPa).
(d) Decadron (dexamethasone) 10 mg i.v.

172 i. The normal higher density cortical gray matter, well seen in the gyri of the right cerebral hemisphere, is decreased in density and indistinguishable from the subcortical white matter on the left. These findings are subtle, but should be carefully sought in the setting of acute stroke, since infarct size can alter management decisions. Patients with very large infarcts are generally not candidates for

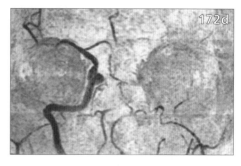

thrombolytic treatment, and should be monitored closely for severe cerebral edema. Of course, the prImary reason for obtaining a CT scan in the setting of suspected infarct is to exclude intracerebral hemorrhage.

ii. The high signal abnormality on diffusion MRI corresponds to the vascular distribution of the anterior and middle cerebral arteries. The posterior cerebral circulation is spared. These findings are most consistent with occlusion of the internal carotid artery, confirmed on MRA (172d).

iii. Diffusion MRI takes advantage of the movement of water as it diffuses by Brownian motion. Application of strong magnetic gradients during acquisition of the MR image, results in overall decrease in magnetization (and therefore signal intensity). Acute cerebral ischemia results in failure of energy-dependent membrane ion pumps, and increased intracellular water. Intracellular water diffuses more slowly than water in the extracellular space, and areas of acute infarct do not lose signal as rapidly as adjacent, uninjured brain. High signal findings on diffusion images can be detected within 1 hour of infarction and last for 2–3 weeks.

173 (d) Decadron. Although steroids are often indicated in patients with *vasogenic* edema, their general usefulness for elevated ICP has not been shown to improve outcome, but can lead to significant side effects including hyperglycemia, sepsis, and increased risk of gastrointestinal bleeding. Rapid administration of osmotic agents such as mannitol (0.5–1.0 g/kg) is the mainstay of treatment of increased ICP and can be used in the patient with cerebral edema and lateral brain displacement from an intracranial mass. The goal for serum osmolality is 310–320 mOsm/L. However, prolonged standing use of mannitol (>48 hr) can lead to rebound increases in ICP if discontinued abruptly. Other effective ways to manage increased ICP include head elevation of 30°, acute hyperventilation to a pCO_2 of 27–30 mmHg (3.6–4 kPa) (resulting in cerebral vasoconstriction), cerebral spinal drainage via a ventricular catheter placement, and barbiturate therapy.

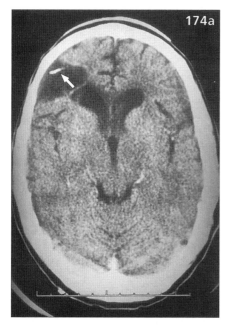

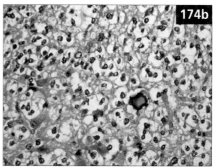

174 This is the CT scan of a 32-year-old male (174a) presenting with right focal motor seizures and the biopsy of the lesion (174b).
i. What does the biopsy show?
ii. What treatment may be helpful in this condition?
iii. What factors may predict a good treatment response?

175 A 49-year-old obese female complains of acute onset of right-sided buttock and leg pain radiating down the back of her leg and into the lateral aspect of her foot. She visits her family physician who discovers an absent ankle jerk and recommends bed rest, a non-steroidal anti-inflammatory agent, and physical therapy. After complying with her physician's advice for 6 weeks with minimal relief, an imaging study is obtained.
    What imaging study is most ideal to evaluate the cause of this patient's pain?

174 i. The biopsy (**174b**) shows the typical appearances of an oligodendroglioma demonstrating the characteristics 'fried egg' appearance. The cells have sharp borders without processes, clear cytoplasm and round uniform central nuclei. In addition there is a fleck of calcium, shown clearly on the CT scan (**174a**, arrow), which is another characteristic of these tumors.

ii. It is now accepted that these tumors are particularly chemosensitive and have shown 75% responses rates to a combination of procarbazine, CCNU and PCV.

iii. Young age, good performance status, extent of surgical resection, loss of heterozygosity on chromosomes 1p/19q.

Oligodendrogliomas are relatively uncommon tumors accounting for about 5–10% of primary brain tumors. They usually occur in young and middle-aged adults and present with seizures, focal neurologic deficits, raised ICP, or combinations of these symptoms and signs. They are occasionally multifocal. Intratumoral calcification is common. They may be low grade or high grade (anaplastic) and are frequently amenable to surgical resection because they occur in non-dominant frontal and temporal lobes. They have a better prognosis than ordinary gliomas because they are chemosensitive. Recently, molecular genetic analysis has shown that patients with anaplastic oligodendrogliomas who have deletions of chromosome 1p/19q have a median survival time for low grade oligodendrogliomas of >10 years.

175 While there are several radio-graphic studies that are commonly employed in evaluating disc disease, including myelogram, CT, and combination of CT with myelography, minimally invasive MRI generally provides the highest yield. In cases where MRI is contraindicated (e.g. cardiac pacemaker, and so on) or when clarification of MRI is necessary, the aforementioned techniques may be supplemented. Routinely, nonenhanced sagittal and axial T1- and T2-weighted images are obtained through the region of interest (**175a** [arrow = herniated disc, arrow head = anteriorly displaced right S1 nerve root, short arrow = thecal sac]; **175b** [arrow = L5/S1 disc]). Gadolinium enhancement is preferable in recurrent post-discectomy symptoms in evaluating the presence or absence of ectopic tissue compressing the nerve root. This may be scar tissue (which enhances) or recurrent disc. One must be aware that a significant percentage of asymptomatic individuals have varying degrees of disc herniation on MRI.

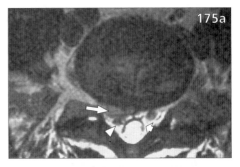

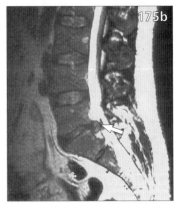

176 With regard to the patient in 175:
i. The appropriate imaging study reveals a large paramedian L5/S1 herniated nucleus pulposis. Is this consistent with the patient's history and physical examination?
ii. What is the accepted standard of care in the treatment of this woman?

177 These three figures (177a–c) show characteristic lesions of a specific neurogenetic disease.
i. Identify the lesions.
ii. What is the diagnosis and typical clinical and pathologic features of this disease?
iii. What is the inheritance pattern?
iv. Is there a DNA test available to confirm the clinical diagnosis?

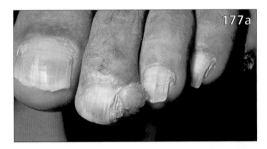

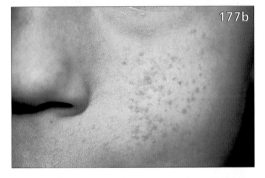

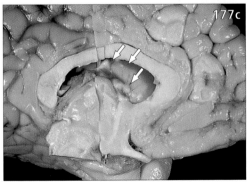

176 i. The patient's classic radiculopathy is in a S1 myotomal distribution. In the lumbar spine, nerve roots exit the intervertebral foramen under the pedicle of the more cranial vertebral level (i.e. the S1 nerve root exits the L5/S1 intervertebral foramen). As the disc space is just inferior to the foramen,

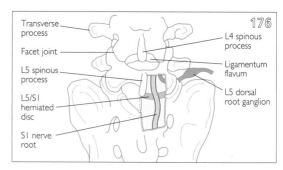

the L5 nerve root has already exited the spinal canal and thus a central or paracentral disc compresses the S1 nerve root (**176**). A far-lateral disc herniation, however, compresses the exiting nerve root at that level (i.e. a far-lateral L5/S1 disc impinges upon the L5 nerve root).

ii. As the majority of disc herniation regress spontaneously, isolated pain should be treated conservatively with non-steroidal anti-inflammatory agents and physical therapy. The issue of bed rest is controversial, as many clinicians now associate persistent pain with muscular atrophy due to bed rest. Pain persisting for >6–12 weeks, or a motor deficit, requires more aggressive treatment. The current standard of care is microsurgical discectomy, which, in appropriately selected patients, can significantly improve radiculopathy in the majority of cases. Complications, including infection, CSF leak, and nerve root injury occur in <5% of cases. There is a 5–10% recurrence rate, either at the same level, or more commonly, at adjacent levels.

177 i. The lesions seen in the figures are a subungual fibroma (**177a**), facial angiofibroma (**177b**) and subependymal nodules or tubers (**177c**, arrows). The brain MRI showed cortical tubers.

ii. This patient has TSC. TSC is a genetic disease that presents with abnormalities of the skin (hypomelanotic macules, shagreen patches, facial angiofibromas, subungual fibromas), brain (cortical tubers and subependymal nodules), kidney (angiolipomas and cyst), heart (rhabdomyoma and arrhythmias). Seizures are a very frequent finding and at least 50% of patients have developmental delay or mental retardation.

iii. The inheritance pattern is autosomal dominant. The offspring of an affected individual are at 50% risk of inheriting the TSC gene. Two-thirds of cases represent new mutations. Variable expression is common.

iv. There is no commercially available DNA test. Molecular testing is available on a research basis only. There are two genes known to cause TSC. The *TSC1* gene at chromosome 9q34 and the *TSC2* gene at chromosome 16 are each responsible for about 50% of the cases. Some sporadic cases probably involve another unknown gene.

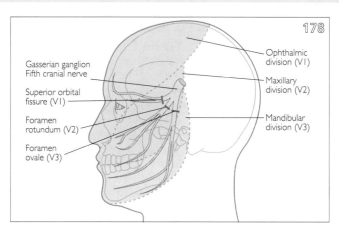

178 A 68-year-old male with a 2-month history of paroxysmal sharp and shooting pain in the mandibular distribution of his left face (178) has been treating his pain with 1 g of acetaminophen every 4 hours, with no significant improvement. His pain is worsened while eating, and he has lost 8 kg (17.8 lb) over the past 2 months.
i. What is the optimal medical management of this patient?
ii. When are surgical options entertained?

179 This 35-year-old female presents with increasing headaches.
i. What does the MRI (179) show?
ii. What surgical approaches are available?
iii. What anatomical landmarks are important in approaching this lesion?
iv. How can access to the tumor be increased?

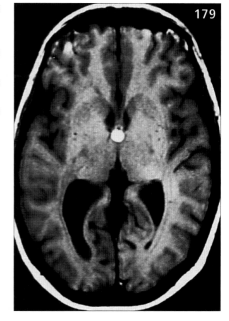

178, 179: Answers

178 i. The described patient exhibits classic symptoms of TGN. While acetaminophen is a well-tolerated general anti-pyretic and pain relieving agent, it is not a useful first-line drug in the management of TGN. Carbamazepine, introduced by Blom in 1962, provides adequate pain relief in close to 70% of patients, and is generally well tolerated. In fact, if 600–800 mg/day is tolerated with no significant pain improvement, the diagnosis of classical TGN is questioned. The dose can slowly be escalated to 1200 mg/day. Baclofen is a second-line drug used in conjunction with carbamazepine. It is particularly useful in patients who cannot tolerate high doses of carbamazepine due to its sedative effects. Pimozide, an anti-psychotic agent used primarily in the treatment of Tourette's disorder, can be used in patients who cannot tolerate carbamazepine. Intravenous phenytoin may be used for patients who cannot open their mouth due to severe pain, as well as patients who are in status trigeminus (recurrent tic-like spasms triggered by innocuous stimuli). Other medications useful in the management of TGN include valproate, clonazepam, and amitriptyline.

ii. Surgical therapy is indicated once a trial of several medications at therapeutic doses have failed, and/or the patient is intolerant to the commonly used drugs at the appropriate doses. Prior to the introduction of effective medical or surgical treatment, suicide was often the only means of cure.

179 i. The MRI shows a colloid cyst in the third ventricle.

ii. The are four basic approaches to colloid cysts: (1) transcortical, transventricular; (2) transcallosal; (3) stereotactic aspiration; or (4) endoscopic. In general the transcallosal approach is favored when the ventricles are small, whereas the transcortical transventricular approach is used when the ventricles are enlarged. Two factors are associated with unsuccessful stereotactic aspiration: small size and hyperdensity (suggesting increased viscosity) on CT scan. A subfrontal approach either subchiasmatic, optico-carotid or through the lamina terminalis may also be used to approach the anterior third ventricle.

iii. The anatomy at the foramen of Monro is important. The choroid plexus passes forward in the choroidal fissure to the foramen of Monro where it converges with the thalamostriate vein that approaches from a more lateral position in a groove between the thalamus and more anterior caudate. The septal and caudate veins approach from anterior.

iv. Access to a colloid cyst in the third ventricle can be achieved interforniceal, which is better suited for lesions in the mid and posterior third of the third ventricle, or through the foramen of Monro. The foramen may be enlarged anterior–superiorly or using a subchoroidal approach posteriorly. The tela choroidea is opened along its medial border, avoiding potential injury to the thalamostriate vein.

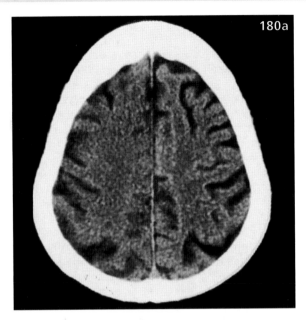

180a

180 A 61-year-old male with poorly controlled hypertension presents to the emergency department with a dense left hemiplegia, a left homonymous hemianopsia, and dysarthria. These symptoms began acutely 90 minutes ago.

i. What is the most appropriate imaging study to obtain at this point?

ii. The head CT shows subtle effacement of the sulci in the right hemisphere (**180a**). The patient's blood pressure is 200/120 mmHg (26.7/16 kPa). His blood glucose is 13.9 mmol/L (250 mg/dl). His body temperature is 38.5°C (101.3°C). What is the most appropriate therapy for this patient?

iii. Assume that this patient's symptoms started 5 hours ago. How does this change your management?

iv. Assume that the patient awakened with these symptoms. He went to bed feeling well 8 hours ago. On examination, you discover that he is in new-onset atrial fibrillation. What is the role of heparin in this situation?

v. How aggressively should his hyperglycemia and hyperthermia be treated?

vi. The patient does well and it is time for him to be discharged to rehabilitation. What is the most appropriate treatment for the secondary prevention of stroke?

180 i. Therapy for acute stroke depends upon whether or not the stroke is hemorrhagic or ischemic. A non-contrast CT scan is the most sensitive radiographic test for detecting acute blood and should be obtained emergently in all patients with the diagnosis of stroke (180a). Infusion CT, or CTA, can also be done on an emergent basis to diagnose large vessel (carotid, MCA, vertebral, or basilar artery) stenosis or thrombosis, which could influence acute management. DWI is now widely available for imaging acute stroke. DWI abnormalities appear shortly (minutes) after stroke onset and persist for only a few weeks after the acute event. DWI is therefore helpful in differentiating acute and chronic changes on imaging studies and should be obtained when possible. Acute stroke therapy should not be delayed, however, in order to obtain a DWI study, unless the diagnosis of stroke is unclear.

ii. The only treatment proven to improve outcome following acute ischemic stroke is thrombolysis. For patients that present within 3 hours of stroke onset, administration of i.v. t-PA at a dose of 0.9 mg/kg is the gold standard of care. The evidence for the benefits of t-PA in acute stroke comes from the NINDS t-PA study. In this study, 26.5% of patients treated with placebo and 42.7% treated with t-PA had complete or nearly complete recovery at 3 months, which correlates to an absolute benefit of 12% and a relative benefit of ~40% in favor of t-PA. The ECASS, however, failed to show a benefit to t-PA administration, which is likely to be related to the fact that t-PA was administered within a 6-hour time window in the ECASS studies. A study of i.v. t-PA in the 3–5 hour time window, the ATLANTIS trial, also failed to show a benefit of t-PA when given later than 3 hours after stroke onset.

In all of the above studies, the use of aspirin and heparin were prescribed for 24 hours following t-PA administration. In the NINDS, ATLANTIS, and ECASS II studies, the blood pressure was also aggressively managed to keep the systolic <185 mmHg (24.7 kPa) and the diastolic <100 mmHg (13.3 kPa). The benefits of t-PA in the NINDS study were independent of stroke subtype. One year follow-up of the original cohort of patients suggests that patients with moderate neurologic deficits (NIHSS score = 10–20) may benefit most.

In all studies of thrombolysis for acute stroke to date, therapy has been associated with a significant increase in the risk of ICH. In the NINDS study, the risk of symptomatic ICH was 6.4% in patients treated with t-PA and 0.6% in patients who received placebo. The only independent predictors of the risk of hemorrhage in this study were the severity of stroke and early CT signs of ischemia. Older patients with severe strokes seem particularly at risk of hemorrhage. The NINDS study, as well as subsequent studies, have shown an association between hyperglycemia and the risk of ICH following thrombolysis, although no data exist to show whether the risk can be decreased with aggressive glucose control.

It should be noted that patients who present with severe stroke and early CT signs of ischemia generally have a poor outcome following stroke. While t-PA may be associated with an increased risk of hemorrhage in these individuals, there is still an overall relative benefit to t-PA administration. The patient presented above has a poor prognosis based on the fact that he has a severe stroke and early CT signs of ischemia. Neither of these findings are absolute contraindications to t-PA administration, although they do increase the likelihood of hemorrhage. His hypertension, however, is an absolute contraindication to t-PA use and must be treated to the blood pressure goals outlined above prior to administration of t-PA. Intravenous labetalol, which is both an alpha- and a beta-adrenergic blocker, is easily titrated and the drug of choice for treating hypertension in acute stroke.

iii. Since >3 hours have elapsed since symptom onset, this patient is not a candidate for i.v. t-PA. A recent study (PROACT), however, showed that patients with occlusion of the proximal MCA (M1) could benefit from intra-arterial thrombolysis if started within 6 hours of symptom onset. The diagnosis of an M1 occlusion can be made non-invasively in the emergency department by TCD or CTA. Unfortunately, the fibrinolytic drug used in the PROACT study, pro-urokinase, has not been approved for use. Therefore, intra-arterial thrombolysis with another lytic agent should be considered as an option for therapy, but is not a gold standard of care.

The IST and the CAST both showed that aspirin at the time of presentation with stroke can decreases the risk of recurrent stroke and death. Based on these two studies, 10 deaths and recurrent strokes will be prevented for every 1000 stroke patients treated with aspirin. The benefit of aspirin seems to be greater the sooner it is given after stroke onset. The dose of aspirin for acute therapy is unclear; it was 160 mg in CAST and 300 mg in IST. In the United States, aspirin is supplied as either an 81 or 325 mg tablet.

Heparin has been used in acute stroke for years despite the lack of data showing any benefit to administration. The IST showed that heparin decreased the risk of recurrent ischemic stroke by 0.9% in the first 2 weeks after presentation, but this decrease was offset by a 0.8% increase in hemorrhagic stroke. In the end, heparin did not decrease the risk of stroke or death. The TOAST also failed to show a benefit to anticoagulation in acute stroke; it did not decrease the risk of recurrent stroke or death and did not decrease the amount of disability experienced by patients who received this low molecular weight heparinoid. Based on these two studies, it appears that heparin is of no benefit to the average stroke patient.

iv. Long-term anticoagulation is undeniably the appropriate therapy for stroke prevention in patients with atrial fibrillation. When to start anticoagulation after acute stroke in patients with atrial fibrillation, however, is not clear. It was long believed that the risk of recurrent stroke in patients with atrial fibrillation was quite high and necessitated immediate anticoagulation. Based on recent prospective studies, however, it appears as if the risk of stroke recurrence in atrial fibrillation was overestimated.

In TOAST, the overall risk of recurrent stroke was 1.2% in the first 7 days; in patients with a presumed cardiac source of embolism, the recurrence rate was 1.6% in placebo treated patients, and not significantly reduced by anticoagulation. In IST, the risk of recurrent ischemic stroke among patients with atrial fibrillation over the first 2 weeks was 2.8% in those receiving heparin and 4.9% in those who were not anticoagulated. While the decrease in recurrent ischemic stroke was statistically significant, the benefit was negated by an increase in hemorrhagic stroke; overall, there was no decrease in stroke or death among patients with atrial fibrillation who were

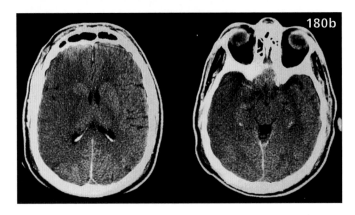

treated acutely with heparin. Therefore, it probably makes sense to wait a few days prior to anticoagulation, especially in patients with large hemispheric strokes (**180b**), since such strokes are often associated with cerebral edema, which may be associated with an increased risk of hemorrhagic conversion.

v. Hyperglycemia in the immediate post-stroke period is associated with increased morbidity and mortality. This risk seems to be limited to patients with large vessel and cortical infarcts. Hyperglycemia is also associated with an increased risk of spontaneous hemorrhagic conversion. While aggressive glycemic control has not been studied in acute stroke, it seems reasonable to normalize the glucose immediately after stroke.

Hyperthermia in the immediate post-stroke period is also associated with increased morbidity and mortality. The detrimental effects of fever are greatest in the first 24 hours following stroke. Increasing brain and body temperature increases the metabolic demands of the brain, although there may be other mechanisms by which hyperthermia exerts its detrimental effects. The benefits of aggressive maintenance of normothermia in acute stroke have not yet been studied, but it makes reasonable sense to use anti-pyretics in the first days after stroke onset.

vi. In order to choose the most appropriate therapy for the secondary prevention of stroke, the pathophysiology of the stroke must be understood. Therapeutic options include anti-platelet agents (aspirin, clopidogrel, ticlopidine, dipyridamole), anti-coagulants (warfarin, low molecular weight heparin), angioplasty, and surgery (CEA and EC–IC artery bypass).

Aspirin remains the gold standard for secondary stroke prevention; meta-analyses show that daily aspirin use decreases the risk of recurrent stroke, MI, or vascular death by approximately 15–20%. The most effective dose of aspirin is unclear, but is likely to be in the range from 50–325 mg daily; Europeans tend to use lower doses than Americans. In a recent prospective trial of aspirin and CEA, patients randomized to low dose aspirin (81 mg or 325 mg) were less likely to experience stroke, MI, or death at 30 days and 3 months following endarterectomy than patients randomized to high dose aspirin (650 mg or 1300 mg). Aspirin exerts an effect through inhibition of cyclooxygenase-dependent platelet aggregation, but may also be beneficial because of its anti-inflammatory properties. For the aspirin intolerant or for 'aspirin failures' (persons that have recurrent stroke while taking aspirin), the thienopyridines (clopidogrel and ticlopidine) are usually prescribed.

Both clopidogrel and ticlopidine prevent ADP-dependent platelet aggregation and both have been shown to be superior to aspirin in prospective, randomized

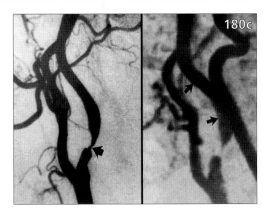

placebo controlled trials. In the CAPRIE study, use of 75 mg q.d. of clopidogrel was associated with an 8.7% relative decrease in primary outcome events (stroke, MI, or vascular death) compared to 325 mg q.d. of aspirin. The absolute benefit of clopidogrel over aspirin was small (0.51%) and probably not clinically meaningful. In the TASS, ticlopidine 250 mg b.i.d. was compared to aspirin 650 mg b.i.d. for the reduction of stroke and death. Ticlopidine use was associated with a 21% relative (3% absolute) decrease in fatal or non-fatal stroke and a 12% relative (2% absolute) decrease in stroke or death in comparison to aspirin. The relatively poor side effect profile of ticlopidine, which includes diarrhea, neutropenia, and thrombotic thrombocytopenic purpura, has resulted in declining use of the drug over past years. The ESPS 2 study showed that sustained release dipyridamole, in combination with aspirin, decreased the risk of stroke (but not the combined risk of stroke and death or the risk of death) in comparison to aspirin alone. The dose of dipyridamole/aspirin used in this study was 200/25 mg b.i.d.

Long-term anticoagulation is indicated for patients with a potential cardiac source of emboli, such as atrial fibrillation or severe cardiomyopathy (ejection fraction <30%). These diagnoses require ECG monitoring and echocardiography. The risk of stroke in patients with atrial fibrillation increases with advancing age, hypertension, and a history of prior TIA or stroke. Women with atrial fibrillation, especially women who take estrogen, also seem to be at higher risk of stroke than men.

Anticoagulation is also advocated for patients with stenosis of the intracranial vessels, based on data from a retrospective study known as the WASIDS. In this study, symptomatic patients with at least 50% stenosis of an intracranial vessel (**180c**) were treated with either warfarin or aspirin at the discretion of their primary physician. The absolute rate of stroke and MI or sudden death were 6.8% lower and 2.9% lower, respectively, in patients treated with warfarin, producing a nearly 50% relative risk reduction in stroke, MI, or vascular death. The diagnosis of large vessel intracranial disease is best done with digital subtraction angiography, but non-invasive studies like TCD, CTA, and MRA can also be used.

CEA is warranted for most patients with symptomatic severe carotid artery disease and for selected patients with asymptomatic carotid disease. The diagnosis can be made non-invasively with carotid duplex. Carotid angioplasty and carotid stenting are now performed more frequently, but the benefits have not yet been proven in a prospective randomized trial. The risk of stroke in patients with carotid stenosis is presumptively related to an increased incidence of thromboembolic events related to the carotid plaque. Early studies of EC–IC bypass in these patients failed to show a benefit. In patients with carotid occlusion, however, stroke can occur due to low blood flow precipitated by relative hypotension. Patients with carotid occlusion at greatest risk for stroke can be identified with PET since the OEF increases in chronically under-perfused tissue. The value of EC–IC bypass in these patients is currently being explored.

Based on the data from the CARE and LIPID studies, it is reasonable to consider 'statin' therapy for secondary stroke prevention in patients with only moderate elevations in cholesterol, as well as those with marked hypercholesterolemia.

Index

Note: all references are to question and answer numbers

Index